W0227859

Background Papers on Industry's Changing Role in Health Care Delivery

WITH CONTRIBUTIONS BY

Karl T. Benedict, Sr., M.D.
  Norton Corporation
John D. Blum, J.D.
  Boston University Health Policy
  Institute
Rick J. Carlson, J.D.

G. H. Collings, Jr., M.D.
  New York Telephone Company

Henry C. Damm, Ph.D.
Karl Bunkelman
  Damm & Associates

Stanley P. deLisser
  National Health Services, Inc.

Henry A. DiPrite
  John Hancock Mutual Life Insurance
  Company

C. Larkin Flanagan, M.D.
James D. Mortimer
Richard B. DiBona
  Continental Bank & Trust Company of
  Chicago

Willis B. Goldbeck
  Washington Business Group
  on Health

William E. Greer, M.D.
Warren Kantrowitz, M.D.
Philip S. White, M.D.
  Gillette Corporation

Thomas Herriman
  Amalgamated Clothing & Textile
  Workers Union

George Himler, M.D.
  W. R. Grace & Company

Alan C. Monheit, Ph.D.
  Boston University Health Policy
  Institute

Sheldon W. Samuels
  AFL-CIO

Mark C. Schofield, M.A.
Richard H. Egdahl, M.D., Ph.D.
  Boston University Health Policy
  Institute

H. A. Sinclaire, M.D.
  Mobil Oil Corporation

Jacob J. Spies
  Employers Insurance of Wausau

Bynum E. Tudor
  R. J. Reynolds Industries, Inc.

SPRINGER SERIES ON INDUSTRY AND HEALTH CARE
NUMBER 3

Background Papers on Industry's Changing Role in Health Care Delivery

Edited by

Richard H. Egdahl

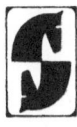

Springer-Verlag New York Heidelberg Berlin

Richard H. Egdahl, M.D., Ph.D.
Center for Industry and Health Care
Boston University Health Policy Institute
53 Bay Street Road
Boston, Massachusetts 02215

Library of Congress Cataloging in Publication Data

Main entry under title:

Background papers on industry's changing role in
    health care delivery.

    (Springer series on industry and health care; no. 3) Presented at a conference
    convened by the Boston University Health Policy Institute in collaboration
    with the Washington Business Group on Health and held in June 1977.
    Bibliography: p.
    Includes index.
    1. Labor and laboring classes—Medical care—United States. I. Egdahl,
    Richard Harrison.   II. Boston University, Health Policy Institute. III.
    Washington Business Group on Health.
HD7102.U4B33   362.1'04'25   77-13611

All rights reserved.

No part of this book may be translated or reproduced in any form without written
permission from Springer-Verlag.

© 1977 by Springer-Verlag New York Inc.

Softcover reprint of the hardcover 1st edition 1977

9 8 7 6 5 4 3 2 1

ISBN-13:978-1-4613-9429-7   e-ISBN-13:978-1-4613-9427-3
DOI: 10.1007/978-1-4613-9427-3

Foreword

Excerpt from Conference Address

One of the most complex and significant social issues facing our nation is reform of our national health system. I am personally committed, and Goodyear Tire & Rubber is committed, to doing everything we can to help improve that system while simultaneously gaining some measure of control over the tremendous rate of cost escalation. I feel very strongly that in the months ahead, business leaders must become actively involved in a concerted effort to strike a balance between our desire to assure the best medical care for all and the reality of doing so at a cost our society can afford.

For the past two years I have been chairman of the Business Roundtable's Task Force on Health and in that capacity have been working closely with the Washington Business Group on Health. Through this exposure and the encouraging results of Goodyear's own cost containment activities, I was asked to serve on HEW Secretary Califano's Advisory Committee on National Health Insurance. This committee, representing a broad spectrum of interests and expertise, will be meeting in cities across the country and will hold hearings in Washington before entering into final discussions with HEW and other administration officials. The result of its work is to be combined with that of the HEW staff in formulating the basis of President Carter's national health insurance proposal.

The committee held its first meeting in Washington on May 20, 1977, and

Secretary Califano's opening remarks made the president's intention completely clear: *"National health insurance (NHI) is a cornerstone of this administration's domestic policy."* He backed that up with the statement that there now exists a national consensus that NHI is desired and needed. No doubt many of us feel this is a bit misleading, since the public can hardly be expected to say no when asked if they would like free medical care—any more than a child would refuse a free lollipop. Such expressions of desire are not necessarily true measures of need, and, as we all know, there is no such thing as free medical care.

To a significant degree, we already have the major elements of a national health system in place. The major private insurance programs, Medicare and Medicaid, the HMO, health planning, manpower, and growing state review programs do in fact combine to produce a national system. Admittedly, it is a system without a central policy, and one that has proven to be only as effective as its interaction with the private sector. One of my primary tasks on the Advisory Committee will be to articulate the contributions of the private sector and to try to establish the principle that any future NHI program must retain the best of the private sector's work while building new initiatives through public–private cooperation. Providing for the health and medical care of the entire nation is simply too large and complex a task for either sector to do alone.

It must also be recognized that, in our system of government, the private sector will always pay 100 percent of health care costs. We have no resources other than those emanating from the private sector. It would be inequitable and foolish to attempt to relieve the private sector of all responsibility for the services it is financing. In fact, we need to create mechanisms for inducing greater responsibility for self-care and greater participation in the cost of care as necessary ingredients of health education and cost containment at all levels of society.

The secretary also identified the major issues on which the administration is seeking the committee's advice, as well as the major principles on which President Carter will base his NHI bill. I am sure you will recognize them. The issues as described by the secretary are:

Access to health care

Inefficiencies in the delivery of services

The need for preventive and primary care

Methods of financing health insurance

The scope of benefits to be covered

The nature and extent of any cost-sharing

Methods of administration, including the role of the private insurance industry

Alternatives for phasing in the plan

The principles on which the president's proposal is to be based are:

Preventive health services, especially for children

Universal and mandatory health insurance to assure equity

Improved efficiency and productivity of the health care industry

Quality control in health care

Consumer participation in the design and operation of NHI

A phase-in of NHI in accordance with the "national priorities of need and feasibility"

I would like to comment briefly on several of these issues and principles. First of all, we can be encouraged by the president's emphasis upon preventive and primary care. For far too long our system has emphasized the most costly curative procedures rather than placing the incentives where they will do the most good for the fewest dollars. One of the items highest on that list, for example, is immunization for children, a program we all can support.

I do become somewhat confused on the undefined issue of equity. When referred to as assurance that everyone will have ready access to quality care in time of need, it appears justified and attainable. If, however, its objective is to see that there is a leveling of services without regard to ability to pay, then I believe it is doomed to failure. There is simply no way that we or any other industrialized society can afford such a system. Basic need should definitely be covered on a universal basis, but I can think of no good reason why one who has the means should be excluded from acquiring a level of care that would otherwise be unavailable. Nor can I think of a reason why taxes should be raised to the astronomical level that would be required to guarantee the most expensive level of care to all.

The principle of efficiency represents the forte of the private sector. I know of no situations—in or out of the health care area—where the government has a record of greater efficiency than the private sector. That is not to say that major improvements cannot or should not be made. Nor is it to suggest that the government is always inefficient. But I do know that there are far more incentives for efficiency when performance is measured by the bottom line rather than by a line item in a trillion-dollar government budget.

Nor can efficiency be attained by the arbitrary establishment of price controls such as those for hospitals in the president's recent message to Congress. A group of us met with Secretary Califano and his staff prior to the issuance of this request and pointed out the futility of such a measure, particularly when the elements of cost, such as labor which represents 55 to 60 percent of their input, were not controlled. I would like to think that we made some impact in that the question of labor cost in the final version was treated separately, and the proposal will quite possibly undergo added changes before final passage.

The quality of service will always be open to question. What is satisfactory today will fall behind with the developments of tomorrow. Certainly we should strive for an improved monitoring system.

The phase-in principle is probably the most important item in the president's list, for it is the cost of an NHI program that has delayed its formulation and implementation to date. The idea of an NHI program is not new and has been with us at least as far back as the Roosevelt era. The deterrent has always been the cost and the belief that this was a price the taxpayer was unwilling to pay. The present administration is fully aware of this, I am sure, but apparently feels that if they can, through the introduction of increased efficiency measures, bring the cost of the services into line, a program can be designed within the stated principles to fit the public's willingness to pay.

This is the area where the Washington Business Group on Health has been most active over the past few years. They have been a source of data compiled from the private sector relating not only to the past and current delivery system, but also to the supporting costs. While this is purely an assumption on my part, I feel the acceptance of reality that this has brought about has contributed to an understanding that, not only from an administrative standpoint but also from a cost standpoint, a program of this magnitude must be phased-in to avoid utter chaos.

One other point that should be mentioned is that, to the best of my knowledge, the question of the capital cost has yet to be adequately addressed. And this is a big one. The majority of hospitals and medical centers are a part of the communities in which they are domiciled. Their capital needs are largely provided for through local fund drives, and many local people take great pride in volunteering their service in support of the work of these institutions.

I lived for a number of years in England under their national health service system and can personally testify that this spirit of personal giving of time and money does not exist to the same degree when health services become the sole responsibility of the state. Thus, any system devised for the United States must, if we are to avoid excess capital cost on an ongoing basis, provide for the retention of the private citizens' enthusiasm and support of their local institutions. Also, if the president's overall program of balancing the budget without undue tax penalties is achieved, an NHI program will have to replace other programs or be phased in over a period of years to coincide with higher tax revenues resulting from increased gross national product. This is a tall order, and there is much work to be done before the final draft is submitted.

There are a number of steps that the nation's industries can take that will, based on our experience at Goodyear, have a positive impact upon costs without in any way diminishing benefits for employees. *The underlying purpose of our activities is to reduce waste so that our health care dollars can be applied to the areas of greatest need.* We have six of our managers serving on various health systems agency (HSA) committees covering activities in the Akron area, and we are similarly involved with HSAs in other areas where we have major payrolls. Between August 1974 and February 1977, the HSA in Akron reviewed $142 million worth of hospital proposals for expansion and other capital outlays in Summit and Portage Counties. The agency approved

$62 million, but rejected $80 million of the proposed spending as being inappropriate. The rejected proposals included one for a whole new 250-bed hospital that would have cost $24 million. The HSA studied the number of hospital beds already available and found it adequate, possibly even excessive. And few homes in the proposed location were more than twenty minutes away from existing hospitals.

I saw an estimate recently that, out of 930,000 hospital beds in the United States, somewhere between 50,000 and 100,000 are surplus—or, to put it in the terms of a production organization, "excess capacity." Others feel that the total may be even greater. It costs about $60,000 these days to provide one new hospital bed, and about half that amount each year to maintain it. With costs like that, any expansion proposals deserve very sharp scrutiny. In one of our cases in Akron, outlays of $14 million in capital will be saved over the next ten years because of active involvement by the HSA and the business community in the expansion process of Akron General Hospital. And the hospital is not forfeiting anything it really needs.

Another way that we are involved at Goodyear is in supporting peer review programs, wherein doctors seek ways to contribute to health care cost control. An example is the number of days that patients need to be kept in hospitals for specific kinds of treatment. Under enabling legislation passed in 1972, HEW has started about 100 of these local professional standards review organizations on a more or less trial basis. Goodyear has funded programs in Akron and in Freeport, Illinois, and we are exploring the feasibility of similar support at some of our other plant locations.

I want to conclude by reemphasizing the importance of ongoing personal and corporate commitment to involvement in these difficult issues. The final shape of NHI may not be as we would like it, but it will be a lot better than if we had not participated.

I can attest that you can be heard. On March 16, 1977, eleven other chief executive officers and I met for an hour and twenty minutes with Secretary Califano—the first time any HEW secretary had met with non-health industry business leaders solely to discuss health policy issues. We did talk about the pending hospital cost control legislation, and we did make clear our opposition to any form of price controls such as the arbitrary 9 percent cap on inpatient care revenues. But more importantly, we exchanged views on the widest possible variety of health care issues. We found that we shared a common concern for the massive waste caused by today's malpractice situation; he was surprised and pleased by our support for health planning; we were glad to hear of his commitment to immunization, community health centers, and mental health.

In response to questions raised during that meeting, the Washington Business Group on Health, under the leadership of Bill Goldbeck, quickly prepared a working paper called *A Private Sector Perspective on Health Care Costs*. This document describes numerous cases of business, often in cooperation with labor and providers, proving that the private sector can make major progress on cost containment while often improving the quality of care. The input of more that seventy companies—acquired in four separate meetings

held in Chicago, New York, and Washington within a two-week period—
provided the basis of the working paper.

I would be remiss if I finished without reiterating my appreciation for the
willingness of Dick Egdahl to direct the resources of this impressive Health
Policy Institute at Boston University to the interaction between industry and
the health sector. This represents a real challenge to us, the business leaders.
We represent the economic strength, managerial capacity, and technical expertise needed to work with the providers and with government to improve the
health care system so that all our people benefit without causing financial
chaos.

June 3, 1977   Charles J. Pilliod, Jr.
                                                Chairman of the Board
                                                Goodyear Tire & Rubber Company

Preface

This volume in the Springer Series on Industry and Health Care arose from a conference on industry-sponsored health programs held in June 1977. The conference was convened by the Boston University Health Policy Institute and attended by corporate and labor union leaders, specialists in the planning, financing, organization, and evaluation of health care, and by physicians and administrators actually delivering health care in corporate settings. Working in a newly emerging field which has as yet no continuous, focused source of information, but which grows in importance daily as calls for changes in our nation's health care system become more urgent, these specialists from diverse backgrounds met to begin to exchange information and viewpoints and to begin to develop the basis of policy options for the future.

Private industry has long been involved in health care, but traditionally in a peripheral, rather passive way. Whether sitting on hospital boards in the spirit of civic duty or expanding the coverage of health insurance benefit packages, both management and labor have often appeared to suspend critical judgment on the actual delivery of care. That role is rapidly changing. Management is analyzing current practices for evidence of the relative payoffs of alternative in-house health programs, and is scrutinizing the cost of insurance claims. Labor is assessing the damage to paychecks and other perquisites from rapidly rising costs for health care benefits. Experiments in corporate health care programs have begun, ranging from the simple but rather recent inclusion of mental health care coverage in benefit packages, through delivery of increased primary health care services in corporate clinics, to the provision of comprehensive prepaid health care sponsored by corporations.

These changes are significant. They mean that management and labor will be increasingly heard in the accelerating national debate over health care. They mean that industry will be watching and participating in the evolution of national health policy and will, in turn, be carefully watched by public policy-makers and by everyone with an interest in how health care for our nation's citizens is financed and delivered. Indeed, private corporations may be, by virtue of their capital resources, purchasing power, and managerial expertise, the most effective change agents available to bring costs under control and revitalize the market in health care.

To assist in this process—to allow industry to hear and be heard in the national debate on health policy, the Boston University Health Policy Institute is organizing, in collaboration with the Washington Business Group on Health, a series of working conferences on industry's changing role in the delivery of health services. From these and other activities will emerge the Springer Series on Industry and Health Care: four monographs a year of health policy analysis synthesizing conference discussions and other special research, and two volumes a year of background papers for each of the conferences prepared by selected participants with special expertise or experience to report.

This first volume of background papers explores industry's varying roles as a provider of health services. Future volumes in the Springer Series will probe the problems and prospects of industry's involvement—the potential of prepaid health plans, the design and administration of employee benefit packages, industry's involvement in community health planning, the nature of industry and union decision-making with regard to health care programs, the impact of those programs on consumer welfare and on our nation's economy— and will further analyze the flawed market in health care, where competition often fails and market incentives and information are inadequate to allow consumers to make informed choices and to receive care of determinate quality at a predictable price.

We at Boston University Health Policy Institute are grateful to the Robert Wood Johnson Foundation for assisting us in holding these conferences, to the Washington Business Group on Health for their collaboration, and to the contributors, whose papers are the book. The spirit of cooperation underlying the contributions and the willingness to share information in the conference lend credence to a conclusion reached recently by the President's Council on Wage and Price Stability:

> Industry and labor appear willing to begin the long and arduous task of reforming the health care delivery system in a way which will ultimately benefit all society because they recognize that such change, in the end, will be in their own self-interest.

Boston
July 1977

Richard H. Egdahl
Series Editor

Diana Chapman Walsh
Assistant Editor

Contents

MODELS

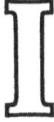

A Corporation's Experience with Independent Practice Association HMOs*

Jacob J. Spies

1

The Employers Insurance of Wausau viewpoint on the individual practice association (IPA) model of HMO is rather unusual, because our company is both an organizer and a purchaser of this type of plan. We have organized and we help administer and coordinate plans at various locations in Wisconsin—Wausau, Green Bay, Milwaukee, Eau Claire, Chippewa Falls—which now involve over 30,000 enrollees, 36 hospitals, and more than 1,500 physicians. We have also purchased this plan for our own employees and their families based in these Wisconsin areas—over 5,100 in all.

A Short History of the Employers of Wausau IPA-HMO

On January 1, 1972, we set into operation an experimental pilot program, the North Central Health Plan, at Wausau, Wisconsin, involving the following participants:

*Copyright 1977 by Employers Insurance of Wausau. All rights reserved.

Marathon County (Wisconsin) Medical Society: initially involving seventy-nine of the society's eighty members, with the plan's activity representing about 5 percent of their patient load

Wausau Hospitals, Inc: two modern, fully equipped hospitals with 407 beds, staffed by over 900 professional and support personnel

Employers Insurance of Wausau: providers of financial resources, administrative and coordinating functions, computer and insurance services

Enrollees: about 3,400 people, consisting of Employers of Wausau employees and their dependents; the North Central Health Plan has since been expanded to include over 16,000 enrollees.

Actually, planning for this experiment had gotten underway as early as 1968. And many years before that, a resolve to develop a new and better approach in group health protection had begun to take form in the minds of a number of our executives, including our former presidents, C. F. Schlueter and T. A. Duckworth. The latter has long been active in local, state, and national health planning activities and became keenly aware of the need for new, more effective and more cost-stabilizing concepts, particularly when he served as chairman of the Wisconsin Advisory Council for Comprehensive Health Planning, and as president of the Wisconsin Regional Medical Program.

Today's health care costs—nearly $140 billion for 1976—are over four times the total 1960 cost. In the fiscal years 1950 through 1976, health care expenditures soared from 4.5 percent to around 9 percent of gross national product. Those in our company who helped conceive and develop our pilot IPA-HMO were mindful in the 1960s that health care costs were then climbing twice as fast as the overall cost of living. The projections at that time had our planners extremely concerned, for they realized that as the health care segment of our economy began to approach 10 percent of GNP, as it is now doing, a factor that could be called "regeneration" would enter the picture.

Economists generally agree that when a segment of GNP reaches the 10 percent level, its effect upon other segments of the economy becomes so powerful that it creates a focal point around which the economy tends to revolve. That particular segment "regenerates" itself because other segments start feeding it and become more dependent upon it, and this forces additional growth that could be unstoppable. This was and continues to be one of the reasons why mounting health care costs are of such major concern.

Our objective in the late 1960s was to create a program that would provide broader medical benefits for a comparable premium dollar, and help to stabilize health care costs. We knew that this could only be achieved through a more effective system of cost controls than we had yet been able to devise. In developing our experimental plan, we studied all traditional as well as recently emerging health care systems. With the help of medical communities around the country, we strove to create a new approach that would combine the strongest features of existing systems with some new concepts of our own, which we believed would result in a better and more universally accepted plan. Our aim was to develop a prepaid plan, but one that would preserve the traditional fee-for-service concept and would not require physicians to join a single medical group. We were guided in our efforts by the estimate that only about one-fourth of the nation's physicians were interested in a prepaid group practice or closed-panel type of plan.

Employers Insurance of Wausau has been deeply involved in the nation's health care system since our company's founding in 1911. We actually did not enter the accident and health field until about 1945, but medical care has always been involved in many lines of coverage that we write, including Workmen's Compensation, public liability, and automobile insurance. Thus, the way in which medical care is financed, delivered, and regulated has great impact upon our company, and we were strongly determined to explore every new concept in health care delivery. We spent five years in our explorations. With the help of our policyholders, medical consultants, physicians, institutional providers, and an interested and cooperative local medical society, we set about to put together a plan that would retain the fee-for-service system, that would allow continuation of all variations of physician practice from solo to clinic, and most importantly, that would have the potential for producing the favorable results achieved by the closed-panel type of HMO, particularly in reducing hospital utilization.

Incentives were built into our pilot plan for all involved to hold down costs. These incentives were balanced with others that were designed to promote rapid and complete recovery through quality health care services. Our experimental plan had an intentionally limited enrollment. We felt that we had to begin with a group whose exact extent of previous coverage was known, and who could be experience-rated through use of the considerable data that had been accumulated. That is why the North Central Health Plan was initially limited to 3,400 people—our own Wausau employees and their dependents.

After more than half a year of encouraging experience with this pilot plan, we proceeded to refine and improve some of its features in preparation for expanding it to other groups in the Wausau area, and later to other Wisconsin communities. Following are some of the basic elements of our plan as it has evolved and is still evolving under the name we call it today, the Health Protection Plan.

The Health Protection Plan—What It Is and How It Works

The plan provides complete coverage for all inpatient and outpatient care. The only major limitation is an annual $50 deductible on over-the-counter prescription drugs. The patient management concept is emphasized by providing benefits for all variations of hospital confinement, including self-care and extended care, plus nursing home care and home care. Preventive care is a major element, because full outpatient health maintenance coverages must be provided if care is to be delivered at the appropriate level, in keeping with the medical needs of the patient. Coverage for preventive care includes immunizations and routine physical examinations as well as office visits, diagnostic testing, and medical eye examinations. The frequency of routine physical examinations is controlled by a schedule developed on the basis of age. A sophisticated health education program is also built into the plan and serves as the real basis for preventive health care, stressing such subjects as weight control, smoking, physical exercise, and hypertension.

The premium, which is paid by the policyholder, is divided into two funds, the physicians' and the general fund, from which charges are paid on a fee-for-service basis. The physicians' fund includes payment of all professional fees of both participating and nonparticipating physicians, the latter being doctors to whom patients are referred under the plan. The general fund covers other charges such as hospital, dentistry, and prescriptions. While the insurer bears the risk of deficits in the general fund, the risk involving the physicians' fund is shared fifty-fifty by physicians and insurer—or, in the case of the Wausau plan, the risk is covered totally by the physicians. In return, the physicians receive any surplus generated in the physicians' fund, for "keeping people well."

In the course of a year, only 90 percent of the physicians' charges are paid to them; 10 percent is held as a hedge against the possibility of a future deficit. However, the physicians' risk is actually not limited to any dollar amount. The income to the physicians' fund comes from a capitation per enrollee. One hundred percent of any surplus developed in the general fund is passed back to the policyholder in the form of rate adjustments or a cash refund. Originally, surplus was shared equally among policyholders, physicians, and hospitals.

The backbone of cost control is the requirement that all providers sign a contract agreeing to the principles of the plan and guaranteeing their specific fees and charges for a twelve-month period of time. Control is achieved first of all through the usual peer review and utilization review committee which studies the statistical output and also the Certified Hospital Admissions Program (CHAP) which is a part of the plan. All of our various health protection plans use the PAS schedule of average length of stays at the 50th percentile. All plan services are coded, using the AMA's Current Procedural Terminology for treatments and either the H-ICDA or ICDA code structure for diagnosis. These produce a myriad of reports which are used by the peer review committee in its work. Because of the success of the Hospital Certification Program, peer review has evolved primarily into an ambulatory review. Among the fifty separate reports produced by our system and used by the peer review committee are charge and service analysis reports by medical practice and by physician; treatment code reports by practice, by physician, by plan, and interrelated; hospital confinement reports by length of stay, by admitting diagnosis, and by treatment; diagnosis reports by physician, and the treatment rendered within each diagnosis; referral reports; out-of-area reports; family profiles, and physician profiles.

Hospital Certification is a most important element in cost control. Within the hospital concurrent review process (CHAP), the PAS guidelines are strictly adhered to. Physicians requesting extensions must submit their reasons in writing to the peer review committee through the patient care coordinator, who has the responsibility for administering the procedures of the certification process, and who reports to the physician peer review committee. Hospital admissions must also be certified as to necessity. Any physician not adhering to the procedure could end up, after three interim steps, in having the cost of an unauthorized hospital charge deducted from his next payment. He would then, in effect, be paying the hospital charge out of his own pocket. The awareness of physicians that they are bearing part of the risk of deficits in the physicians' fund and the knowledge that overutilization would have a direct effect upon its solvency create an effective cost control factor. While it may take persuasion to get some physicians to accept this sharing of risk, they eventually see it as a visible indication of their desire to help solve the serious problem of soaring health care costs. This is what makes peer review work, for it is an educational and not a punitive process.

Another effective form of peer review is the monthly summary report which each participating physician receives and which indicates precisely, by name, what each physician took out of the fund. The summary highlights several categories of information including the number of patients seen, the average charge made, the average number of services rendered per patient, and the number of office visits, x-rays, and hospital visits. In this way the summary report serves to highlight differences in practice habits and charging habits. Voluntary changes have been made by some physicians, even within certain specialty groups, as a result of the monthly summary. Two areas where significant changes have taken place are therapeutic injections and office visit callbacks.

Health educational efforts are built into the plan and serve as the basis for preventive care. In view of this, and realizing that enrollees have an important role to play in efficient administration of the plan and in cost control, we periodically publish a newsletter to inform and motivate enrollees in the proper use of Health Protection Plan features. Purposes of the newsletter are summed up by the following feature which introduced the first issue to its readers:

IT'S HEALTHY TO KEEP INFORMED

... and that's why this Health Protection Plan newsletter will come your way occasionally, from now on, reminding you of the Plan's basic purposes and procedures.

We hope that our newsletter will help you come to see the Health Protection Plan as a beneficial partnership which includes you ... your dependents ... your employer ... your family physician ... hospital ... clinic ... and your Plan's administrator—all joined in an enterprise for quality health care at the lowest possible cost.

Among other important purposes, our newsletter will:

Remind you about Plan benefits available to you and yours.

Clear up common misunderstandings about your Plan.

> Stress proper use of your Plan, so that overall costs and premiums can be held to a minimum.
>
> Bring you new and timely tips on personal health and safety.
>
> To sum it all up, our newsletter will aim to keep the Health Protection Plan sound and healthy, so that it is better able to protect your health, and that of your dependents.

To encourage questions and suggestions from enrollees, so that we can clear up common misunderstandings and improve routine administration of the plan, we attach a postage-free reader's reply card to each issue circulated. Numerous cards have been received, bringing us questions that we answer either by direct correspondence or in issues of the newsletter. Many positive and appreciative comments about both the newsletter and the Health Protection Plan have been received through this medium.

Results Achieved by the Health Protection Plan

Over 94 percent of our eligible employees are covered under the Health Protection Plan. It was originally offered as a dual-choice option, but has emerged as the health program favored by our Wisconsin employees in those cities where the plan is in operation. Prominent among the reasons for enthusiastic acceptance is the freedom of choice of physician for enrollees and their dependents, with no need to disrupt long-standing patient-physician relationships. The published list of participating physicians has also been influential in bringing some physicians into the plan, as they were motivated to sign contracts of participation after a number of their patients contacted them to ask if they expected to join the plan.

Other factors that help account for the excellent enrollee reaction are guaranteed availability of care and the plan's extremely broad coverage without the usual limitations. Because of this and the health maintenance coverages that are included, patients have much less out-of-pocket expense than they incurred with traditional plans. Administration is totally computerized. The only time enrollees receive a bill is when they receive care out of the service area, either on a referral or emergency basis. There are no claim forms to fill out; patients merely present an identification card and receive whatever care is required.

The concept of preventive medicine is a very popular plan feature. Our company has a periodic physical examination which previously required a certain financial outlay. This entire program has now been absorbed by the Health Protection Plan and we have modified it to meet the examination sequence set up under the plan. The controlled length of hospital stay is also quite favorably regarded by our people.

The response from participating physicians has also been generally enthusiastic. Doctors particularly like the fact that the doctor-patient relationship is preserved, and, as previously observed, the majority of physicians strongly favor the IPA type of HMO over the closed-panel system. Many participating physicians are also convinced that our plan is making a valuable contribution toward the stabilization of health care costs. One hundred percent of the physicians in Wausau are participating in the North Central Health Protection Plan. The same is true in Chippewa Falls and Eau Claire. In Green Bay, all but a few physicians have signed contracts. Nearly 1,000 Milwaukee area physicians are participating in our newest plan, representing over 80 percent of the primary care physicians in that city.

We at Employers of Wausau can look at our IPA experience from an unusual viewpoint that combines developmental and managerial as well as employer-purchaser experience. And we have found that the Health Protection Plan has brought significant benefits to our company, as purchasers of coverage. First, there is no question that our employee relations are very good. Perhaps a negative aspect of this is that since our people have no complaints about our group health program, some have probably been inclined to intensify their criticism of other fringe benefits.

We have found that the plan is easily explainable to our new employees. Another positive effect is that with the reduction in hospital stays, our people do not lose as much time from work. An individual who would have been confined for nine days and is now instead confined for four will perhaps return to work one or two days sooner than could have been previously anticipated. While this is difficult to measure, we do have some evidence that it is taking place, and the cost saved must certainly be credited to the program.

The plan has some disadvantages for the employer that should be recognized. First, since it is such a broad plan, there is a natural tendency for employees to want more and more. Also, some employees would rather have their care provided outside of the service area of a prepaid plan. This is not possible unless a referral is obtained, and frequently, owing to physicians' attitudes on cost containment, referrals are not easily obtained if physicians feel that they are not really necessary.

There is also a potential problem of overuse, which is of course present with traditional programs, but which is possibly more severe with an HMO that is virtually unlimited in coverage. It is necessary to watch continuously the amount of care that is being delivered to any one enrollee, so that potential abuse can be identified early. In our plan, this is achieved through activity audits of the management system. The system produces a quarterly report showing the total activity on the part of a family that exceeds a certain dollar amount. From this, patient profiles are produced on those cases where there is a suspicion of overuse, and our personnel department is then able to follow up by reminding the employee of his responsibilities under the plan.

Another problem we encountered earlier as a purchaser of the plan is the one created by no patient billing, which leaves employees totally in the dark as to the value of plan benefits. Plan administrators solved this in two ways. First, they make sure that each patient gets a copy of the hospital bill, even though it is not a request for payment. Since hospital charges generally represent the most expensive portion of health care costs, this gives employees some idea of these costs and what has been paid in their behalf. The doctor is also sent a copy of the hospital bill so that he understands what charges are being incurred by his patient outside of his or her own billing responsibilities. The patient is also given a copy of the encounter form or route slip that the doctor uses in his office. Since these are precoded and prepriced, the patient then not only sees what the doctor did during this visit and what was charged for the treatment, but sees also the entire listing of the physician's charges for most of the treatments performed.

Finally, each enrolled family is sent a summary of all health services received during the previous calendar year. This report shows the date each service was rendered, the doctor who provided it, the specific type of service, and the charge made. All charges are totalled and the patient then gets some idea of the value of benefits delivered in his behalf. A covering letter from the employer also helps to underline the value of the Health Protection Plan. This summary report has been quite popular; it is an excellent management and personnel tool, and it also performs an audit function, as it makes possible a double check by patient of all charges for the year.

Another HMO feature that might possibly be disadvantageous is the fact that the benefit package is somewhat rigid, and the services offered are largely controlled by the physicians rather than by what the employer might desire to offer his employees. This tends to eliminate part of the employer's prerogatives and bargaining power and could to some extent affect budgetary planning, although this has not posed any direct problem for our company.

We are a nationwide corporation with employees located throughout the country, but we are able to include only Wisonsin-based employees in the Health Protection Plan. Our non-Wisconsin people, who represent about two-thirds of our total work force, are covered under a traditional program which we call the Universal Plan. From some in the latter plan we have had complaints about the inaccessibility of the broader benefit package. To this date we have not differentiated employee contributions for the two programs, but we will probably have to take steps in this direction eventually. This is a situation that must inevitably be faced by many companies as HMOs come into being throughout the country.

All in all, the advantages of the plan for employers seem to outweigh by far the disadvantages. Numerous employer groups have expressed interest, primarily because they are convinced that the plan has the potential for stabilizing and perhaps reducing premium costs. In the five years the plan has been in existence, only one employee group has dropped it—and that was due to its experience-rate level. Over 94 percent of our eligible employees are covered by the Health Protection Plan. The administrators tell us that this fact allows them to require 75 percent participation in those groups to whom they present the plan, and they have been achieving far in excess of that participation.

Comparison of Health Protection and Universal Plans

Since health care costs in some of the Wisconsin cities involved with the Health Protection Plan are representative of some of the higher cost areas throughout the nation, we feel that we can make a valid comparison between

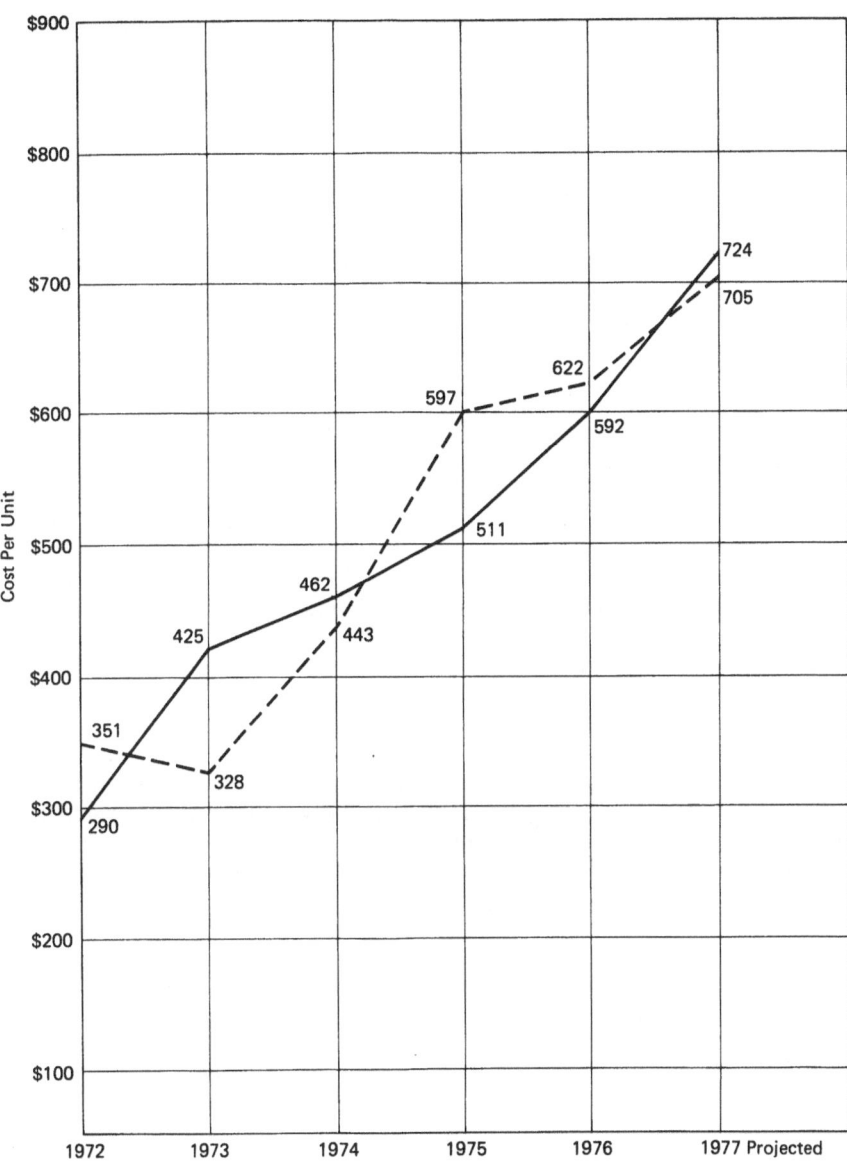

Figure 1.
Health Protection Plan and Universal Plan, 1972–1977. (---) Health Protection
Plan; (___) Universal Plan.

the experience of the one-third of our people within the Health Protection Plan, and the remaining two-thirds covered by the traditional Universal Plan. Costs can be readily compared; figure 1 reveals that the per claim cost per employee is increasing more rapidly under the Universal Plan. While the Health Protection Plan started out at a higher figure, the lines crossed during 1977.

The rapid jump in Health Protection Plan benefit payments between 1973 and 1975 was due in part to the removal of medical controls by the federal government and the introduction at the same time of a rather sophisticated and comprehensive "encounter form" to be used by physicians for all ambulatory _ervices. Use of the latter had the effect of "unbundling" specific groupings of charges and, in essence, of spreading the physicians' charging potential over a broader base. We have since taken steps to make sure that this phenomenon will not happen again, by totally computerizing our actuarial program. We now get monthly updates on pure premium costs and are able to revise our annual premiums for new business on a monthly basis if necessary. We are thus able to reprice our product continuously, based on current costs and utilization.

The continually rising costs of traditional health insurance are based on projected inflationary increases which are to great extent guesswork. However, our extremely responsive and accurate computer system provides management information that enables us to adjust plan costs by specific inflationary increases which are not determined by guesswork. Because of this capability, we are projecting a continually widening differential between the company's Universal and Health Protection Plans in the coming years.

A review of statistical information enables us to pinpoint other specific results thus far achieved by the Health Protection Plan. The average length of hospital stay has been reduced over three days—from 7.4 to 4.3 days. This is a 39 percent reduction in days confined. Since the average length of stay nationally is still close to eight days, this is a particularly significant achievement.

In an attempt to limit "diagnostic only" admissions and to provide more outpatient coverage, we have reduced hospital admissions by close to 10 percent. While this figure does not seem large, it becomes more impressive when you multiply it by the average cost of a hospital stay. It has been estimated that the reduction of each hospital stay by a single day, nationally, would achieve an annual saving of over $3 billion, or about 3 percent of the claim dollar. The national average number of days confined annually per 1,000 people insured is about 1,100 for our mix of participants. Most prepaid plans have been effective in reducing this considerably, and under our program the reduction has been to 469 days.

The statistic that perhaps has more immediate meaning is an overall saving in total health care costs of over 21 percent. Thus, a traditional plan incorporating Health Protection Plan benefits but without its control and incentives would cost 21 percent more than does our program. Generally, the average program provides financing for about 70 percent of a family's annual health care needs, with 30 percent paid out of pocket. Under our plan, out-of-pocket expenses are reduced to 9 percent.

As the plan administrator, we can claim only partial credit for the achievements of the Health Protection Plan. While we gather the statistics and channel the funds, it is the participating health professionals who are the determining factor. Working together, diligently and cooperatively, they have helped to win the way toward the goals we all set for ourselves during those early planning stages in the mid and late 1960s.

Summary of Major Advantages of an IPA-HMO

Following are some of the major advantages of the Health Protection Plan, as revealed by our experience as both an organizer and purchaser of this kind of HMO:

Low start-up costs owing to use of existing facilities; integration with existing physicians' practices; and minimal overhead while waiting for enrollees.

Acceptable to the majority of physicians; surveys indicate that 75 percent of physicians would not accept traditional (cosed-panel) prepaid group practice.

Acceptable to hospitals. Hospitals realize that changes are inevitable and see the plan as an opportunity for gradual change. They are also aware that the plan could affect their income, but they accept it because it enables them to project and plan more accurately for utilization, and shorter lengths of stay enable them to better utilize existing beds.

An opportunity for insurers to continue their role as risk bearers and as administrators of health insurance; it is an opportunity to set up, manage, and control an HMO, rather than merely to support and finance it.

Administration is completely computerized, which helps to ensure accuracy and efficiency. Cost will vary by group, but should generally be about 10 to 15 percent higher than a good major medical plan.

One Enrollee's Experience

As purchasers of the Health Protection Plan for our own Wisconsin employees and their families, we have been pleased to note the gratitude voiced by many of our people. "It's the Cadillac of health insurance plans," is the attitude that is commonly expressed. And for some, the gratitude runs far deeper. In 1973, one of our young Green Bay employees went to his doctor for a routine checkup. Examinations by an internist and a cardiologist revealed a serious heart problem, and a doubtful future if something were not done promptly. "Soon afterward," our employee reported, "some steep bills for medical services began arriving. But the Health Protection Plan came to the rescue and I realized that I had one less thing to worry about. I found that if your doctor refers you to a specialist who is not in the plan—in my case a cardiovascular surgeon—his services are also covered."

Open heart surgery was performed to remove and graft a damaged aorta section and replace an aortic valve—the first time a double heart repair operation of that type was ever performed at Green Bay's Bellin Memorial Hospital. Recovery was long and difficult. Then half a year later, a second open-heart operation was required since the new valve had torn loose and had to be replaced. This meant more drastic costs, and another long and difficult recovery. "I don't know what I'd have done without the Health Protection Plan," our Green Bay employee said. "We probably would have lost our house. My wife and I referred to the plan as our White Knight, because every time we'd get a bill the plan would come to our aid, handling everything with no anxiety for us." Hospital and doctors' bills for the two operations and other services totaled more than $38,000, and time off the job came to nearly six months. We are happy to report that our employee has now been back on the job full-time for nearly two years without further physical problems. He walks two miles a day and plays golf regularly—and we believe that our Health Protection Plan contributed substantially to the happy outcome.

Evaluations by Outside Observers

Perhaps the most significant opinions of our Health Protection Plan are those objective ones of people outside both the plan and our company, who have come to observe. Jack D. Martin, Midwest editor of *Medical Economics*, had this to say in the September 16, 1974, issue of that journal:

> A plan like Wausau's can retain the known advantages of fee-for-service practice while it reaches for the promised advantages of prepaid group practice . . . The Wausau prototype of an "HMO without walls" to a degree resembles groups in other areas where participating physicians work out of their own offices and are paid on a fee-for-service basis from funds collected on prepayment contracts. Unlike most of the others, however, the Wausau HMO serves patients covered by private employers' group insurance rather than patients under government-sponsored programs . . .
>
> The plan's success is credited to the way it combines various elements, none without precedents elsewhere, to satisfy everyone concerned—those who provide, receive, and pay for the services it offers . . . There's almost no doubt that any program of national health insurance Congress enacts will offer incentives to prepaid group practice. The Wausau experience looks like good news for physicians who want to retain traditional doctor-patient initiatives in the face of that trend.

As for cost investment aspects of the Health Protection Plan, the August 20, 1973, issue of *American Medical News* reports:

Employers of Wausau figures its total cash investment, covering all three plans (Wausau, Green Bay, Milwaukee), will come to little more than $150,000. That's less than 2 percent of the investment made by Connecticut General as a result of its health plan involvements.

As with other insurers, Employers does not "own" its plans. Rather, it is a participating co-sponsor, along with local providers and other carriers. In Milwaukee, a citizens advisory group on health care is also involved.

In September, 1975, twenty-five representatives of the U.S. Department of Health, Education, and Welfare came to Wausau to learn more about our plan, having a particular interest in the open-panel or individual group practice feature. Frank Seubold, associate director of the Bureau of Community Health Services for HEW, was quoted in the Wausau, Wisconsin *Daily Herald:* "The plan is . . . one of the older, best established, and best run in the nation . . . It appears to be an eminently reproducible model." Seubold, who is responsible for developing health maintenance organizations, said that HEW sees a big value in an open-panel system because it enlarges the available physicians' resources. He expects to see a rise in open-panel plans throughout the nation, and cited studies showing that HMO participants save from 15 to 30 percent of what they would have had to pay for health care under conventional insurance.

Robert A. Zelten, director of the HMO program for the Wharton School of Business of the University of Pennsylvania, and associate professor of insurance there, was quoted in the March 11, 1976, issue of Wausau's *Daily Herald:*

An HMO with an IPA (individual practice association) is scarce, and good IPAs are even scarcer. A lot of people don't think IPAs can work, but Employers has demonstrated that they can be an improvement over the traditional system.

We know of no IPA plan that compares to the one at Employers in terms of structure, controls and performance.

The preceding facts, figures, advantages, disadvantages, and achievements sum up our corporate experience thus far with the Health Protection Plan variety of an IPA-HMO, as both a developer-administrator and a purchaser of the plan. Employers Insurance of Wausau shares with physicians, hospital administrators, employer groups, insured employees and their dependents, HEW observers, and others a strong enthusiasm and confidence in the program, as well as an optimism about its further potential and its future.

Health—A Corporate Dilemma; Health Care Management—A Corporate Solution

G. H. Collings, Jr.

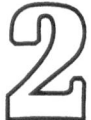

Society requires that business accept responsibility for injuries to employees that result from the job. Yet, when it comes to deciding what this means in specific circumstances, it has not been easy to establish the limits of such responsibility. In fact, over a period of many years these limits have been the subject of endless controversy accompanied by progressive liberalization of benefits for the employee and an increasing accountability for the corporation. New legislation and interpretation of old legislation continue to extend former practices beyond simple financial reparation and payment of medical costs, to include such things as rehabilitation, retraining, and adjustment of job duties to accommodate residual handicaps. Even total career protection and lifetime security have been sought as proper compensation for those hurt at work.

Over the same time period there has been a broadening of what is meant by injury at work, first to include, in addition to physical injury, diseases produced by the work environment (the so-called occupational diseases) and then to include diseases that are not caused by the job but are simply aggravated or adversely affected by the job in some way. The truth of the matter, of course, is that *any* disease in an employee is influenced by the job. In fact, the health of employees who have *no* demonstrable disease in the ordinary sense is also significantly influenced by the job—or any other activity that occupies as much as eight hours out of twenty-four. Consequently, the dividing line between occupational and nonoccupational illness has become increasingly hard to identify, even though the reparations made to or on behalf of the employee may still differ significantly depending on which category is assigned. Part of the corporate health dilemma arises from this incongruous situation. Should the corporation continue to try to maintain the fiction of occupational versus nonoccupational categorization with assignment of responsibility for the former to the corporation and for the latter to the individual? If not, where and how do the responsibilities of the corporation and of the individual interact?

It is also a widely accepted principle that business should take precautions to eliminate hazardous conditions from the working environment. Recently shored up by the Occupational Safety and Health Act and other legislation, this principle has acquired much broader significance in terms of what must be done to meet the requirements of the law. But as was the case with Workmen's Compensation, the impact of these environmental laws is being determined more by interpretations handed down under the law than by the original statutes themselves.

How far should the corporation go in regard to its work environments? Eliminate hazards that are demonstrably injurious, certainly. But what about potential hazards? How far does the corporation go in expenditure of time, money, and effort to evaluate those situations that might *possibly* have an effect on employees? And how significant must the effect be before it reaches the level of concern? The healthy human body can deal with small quantities of chemical, physical, and psychological moieties without apparent damage but not without effect. Is it the employee's responsibility to accept minimal effects as part of what a salary is for, or should the corpoation go further in reducing these apparently innocuous exposures? The truth is, of course, that more and more of what were previously judged to be innocuous turn out to be significant whether they be chemical agents, carcinogens, psychological stresses, or whatever. Furthermore, individual employees vary considerably in their ability to tolerate minor environmental stresses. Is the absolute elimination of all environmental stress required so that the most sensitive employee may work in freedom from any effect?

And then there is the matter of how the environmental stress is to be controlled or eliminated. How much should the worker be expected to actively participate (such for example as in the wearing of noise protection equipment) and how much should the corporation be expected to eliminate the stress, by perhaps costly engineering or other means, so that workers might be passively protected? These matters relating to the work environment also contribute to the corporate dilemma on health.

Yet another area of even greater concern is related to the escalating costs associated with health (or the lack of it)—hospitalization insurance, medical care costs, sick pay, and other health-related benefits provided for employees and their families. In New York Telephone, which is fairly typical of large industry generally, these costs make up about 10 percent of the total wage package, and have been inflating at an increasing rate each year. Last year they were up 25 percent over the year before, having reached a total for the year of $117 million.

In a nutshell, industry is paying for the bulk of the health costs for its employees and their families; these costs are assuming proportions that cannot be ignored by even the most profitable of corporations, and yet industry has not been provided with a participating role in the operation of the health care system. This produces the frustration of accountability without the opportunity for constructive action.

Yet another source of frustration is the fact that in spite of these huge and expanding expenditures, the health of employees seems little if at all better than before. Although our ways of measuring health are admittedly limited, those measures that we do have when applied to the present work force do not show it to have significantly improved mortality, morbidity, or diability.

To summarize, business has acquired health responsibilities that were originally related only to the work environment but which have now expanded to the point of pervading a substantial segment of the total health picture. Yet the corporation is frustrated on many counts by factors that limit severely its capacity to cope with these responsibilities. These factors are that the inherent nature of most of these problems is complex; the present health care system has shown little interest in industry's problems and concerns; and more importantly, the health care system has great capacity to prevent "outsider" intervention which has effectively blocked most attempts by industry to influence established patterns of health care or the efficiency of the health care process.

The businessman is left searching for ways out of this dilemma. This search has produced a variety of attempts to find a solution, varying all the way from complete duplication of the community health care system (as in the Kaiser plan) to minor fiscal constraints and the application of rhetoric.

At New York Telephone over the past few years, we have considered and discarded most of the ideas that have been put forward as being unrealistic or unattractive for one reason or another. In the process, it has become clear to us, however, that the solution must include greater involvement of the corporation in health care and in finding a way to manage the health care process without duplicating the existing system. We are evolving an approach which we call Health Care Management (HCM). It is based on authority provided voluntarily by each employee to manage his health and to serve as his health surrogate. The objective of HCM is to provide a mechanism through which a positive effect on the real health of employees may be achieved while containing health-related costs and optimizing efficiency of the health care system.

Basically, the HCM idea is a very simple one. In essence, it says that if the health of an employee could be managed by competent professionals in the company's medical department in its entirety, it would be possible (within the limits of the circumstances of that particular individual and within the limits of the state of the art of the health sciences) to guarantee that individual the best health for the longest time and to guarantee that the health services delivered would be of the highest quality at lowest cost. Further, the idea says that if a majority of the individuals in an industrial population were managed in this way, the health care of the entire working population could, for all practical purposes, be brought under effective control.

HCM divides logically into three interrelated but conceptually distinct levels. Level I HCM is the management of a specific illness or injury (a case of pneumonia, a broken leg, ureteral colic, congestive heart failure, and so on). Level I management requires a disease orientation and operates within a logic that seeks first a diagnosis and then a therapy designed to eliminate (or cure) the illness. This is what most physicians do best. It is also what most of the medical resources and the health professionals of this country have been prepared to provide. It should not be surprising therefore that Level I functions are commonly mistaken for the *whole* of health care.

However, it will become apparent that the basic HCM theory is viable only if the industrial medical professionals who undertake Level I management are also skilled in the performance of traditional business management functions, and only if the individual employee cooperates fully with these efforts. It follows that delivery of a certain amount of Level I medical care in-house is necessary to initiate and hold the employee in a relationship with the industrial medical professional that will in turn provide the professional with the authority to manage the employee's whole health. However, beyond whatever minimum amount of direct medical care is required to attain that objective (which will obviously vary from employee to employee), delivery of additional Level I medical care in-house is not desirable for a variety of reasons. Management and coordination of the Level I care being delivered is the more pertinent objective.

Level II management is oriented toward the *whole* individual; it includes planning a lifetime health strategy for the individual, guiding health education, periodic health monitoring, applying preventive measures, and overall supervision of the individual's total health care within the context of the lifetime health strategy. HCM logic calls for Level II management to be done exclusively in-house. It is not realistically available from the community, and it requires expertise in preventive and constructive medicine which is most readily provided in-house.

To be successful, Level II HCM requires that the participating employee cooperate fully and conscientiously with the health plan outlined for him by the Level II manager. It is therefore essential that a harmonious relationship with mutual respect and confidence be developed and maintained between the employee and the Level II manager. This will not always happen spontaneously. Consequently, a conscious effort must be made to attract the employee and then to build a relationship that is comfortable and satisfying with that employee. In the HCM program this is referred to as "capturing" the employee, and it is here that Level I and Level II activities become interdependent; a certain amount of Level I medical care must usually be delivered personally by the Level II manager to capture the typical employee.

Level III management deals with population groups and subgroups. It applies the principles of epidemiology and biostatistics to the characterization of a specific industrial population. In the case of HCM, the population is the over 80,000 employees of New York Telephone, approximately half of whom are women and all of whom have definable geographic, demographic, ethnic, economic, occupational, and other characteristics that may have significant bearing on their state of health and on any program such as HCM that attempts to improve that state.

Level III HCM, by study of this employee population and its major subpopulation (those who voluntarily participate in the HCM program), identifies areas of greatest concern and opportunities for greatest achievement and develops specific programs to capitalize these opportunities. Allocations of available resources are then possible to achieve maximum effectiveness. Level III management also concerns itself with evaluation in many forms. There is evaluation of the efficacy of clinical procedures, overall evaluation of the employee population's quality of health and its performance in such matters as productivity, absence, disability, and cost, and also study and evaluation of the HCM machinery itself to strengthen its weak spots and fine tune the whole for more effective operation.

There are a number of ways that an individual employee can begin to participate in HCM. He or she could have heard of the program from a fellow employee or have read about it and decided to come in to inquire for more information. Or, he or she may have been told of the HCM program at the time of a periodic health examination. Or, owing to some illness or injury, the employee may have been coming to the medical department and have already developed a comfortable relationship with one of the doctors who then used that opportunity to introduce the employee to HCM. Or, there may have been other lead-in circumstances including some so subtle that there was little or no conscious awareness on the employee's part of actually joining an organized program. Rather, he or she may simply have willingly accepted an expanding relationship with the medical department, taking advantage of increasing offerings of services that fit in with perceived needs.

Given the foregoing circumstances, the first concern of the Level II manager is to "capture" the individual to be managed. By this is meant to establish a relationship with the employee that will be conducive to voluntary participation with the manager in what the manager has to offer. It is apparent that capturing the patient may not be easy, but it is certainly of sufficient importance to warrant special consideration in the training of nurses and doctors who intend to practice Level II management and in their continuing efforts to improve their own performance in that practice. In essence, the would-be Level II manager needs to become familiar with the intended patient's life, attitudes, and circumstances and insofar as possible to try to place himself in the position of the patient so as to appreciate how best to present HCM in a way that will be responsive to the patient's needs and will be perceived by the patient as attractive.

Furthermore, capture of the patient should not be viewed as a one-time event after which no further attention need be given to the patient-manager relationship. On the contrary, this relationship needs continuing emphasis and conscious, persistent attention to maintain and improve the bonds already established. Probably, "capture and hold" would be a more accurate expression of this requirement for Level II management.

Having captured a patient, or having one in the process of capture, the manager must promptly also give attention to the basic objective, which is to look after this new patient's health. The manager will therefore naturally want to develop the first edition of a lifetime health strategy for this patient, but before he can do that meaningfully, he needs to learn as much as possible about the patient so that he will have an adequate basis for his decisions. In other words, he needs to characterize his patient—is he overweight? Does he smoke? What kind of nutritional background does he have? What are his current activities and Work, family and home situations? Is he prone to allergies? And on and on. Unfortunately, completely characterizing a new patient requires the acquisition, organization, and review of an enormous amount of information—obviously, an impossible task for a single encounter and a task that will probably have to be pursued for quite some time, if not permanently. Nevertheless, a start must be made. Under HCM, that start is called the baseline examination. If no previous medical record is available, the baseline examination must range widely and probe deeply into most aspects of the patient's past and present. If some prior information is available, the baseline examination must summarize the pertinent pieces of that past accumulation, fill in any gaps, and add adequate evaluation of present health. In other words, the baseline examination is a comprehensive process—not a screening examination.

Having carried out a suitable baseline examination, the Level II manager will then want to familiarize himself with the accumulated information and reach appropriate conclusions as to the characteristics of that patient that are pertinent and important to making long-range plans. Of equal importance (or perhaps initially of greater importance) will be the identification of things that are now wrong with the patient's health and what can be done about them. The management of these individual diseases will be primarily a Level I function but the Level II manager needs to recognize the immediate medical problems and provide for their solution in the overall plan.

The overall plan for a patient in HCM is known as the lifetime health strategy. The first version of the lifetime health strategy is developed as a result of the baseline examination and the analysis of the information gained thereby. The lifetime health strategy should not be viewed as a static game plan to be relentlessly pursued, but as a dynamic process undertaken in the beginning, added to or modified as additional information or experience accumulate, improved as new scientific knowledge becomes available, and adapted to the responses of patients generally or more importantly to the response of that individual patient. The important thing is not so much the specific plan at any one point in time as it is the necessity for the manager to keep reassessing the plan in the light of current developments—constantly striving to improve the likelihood of the plan's success.

As part of the lifetime health strategy the manager will make certain recommendations to the patient. Some of these will be individualized for that particular patient; others will be more general and should be included as a part of everyone's lifetime health strategy. Both types of recommendations developed by the manager will be discussed with the patient and an appropriate plan of action involving commitment by the patient will be initiated.

In addition to the recommended measures, the complete lifetime health strategy will make provision for future information acquisition and for the opportunity to revise the strategy. These future update points (that is, periodic health assessments) need to be individualized for each patient. Healthy young adults, for example, may not need another health assessment for three to five years or more, while older patients or those with specific diseases may require an update in six months or less. Of equal importance, the content of the periodic assessment needs to be individualized. The 27-year-old female with no history of early sexual activity who was married at 22 years of age, has no children, and who has had three negative Pap smears since age 22 does not need a repeat Pap smear at every periodic health assessment. This test might will be included, however, for other patients whose risk factors indicate a greater probability of cervical cancer occurrence.

Here is one point where Level II and Level III managements interface. The specific studies done by Level III management to determine the epidemiology of disease in the target population (New York Telephone employees) provide information that makes it possible for the Level II manager to individualize the periodic update plans for each patient. Conversely, the findings from individual patients collectively form the basis for Level III studies.

This is also another point where the dissimilarity between HCM and more traditional occupational health programs is apparent. Traditional programs (executive examinations, periodic examinations, multiphasic screening, and so on) tend to apply the same procedures to all patients at fixed and standardized intervals. HCM's update component attempts to vary both the frequency and the content of examinations to best suit the needs of the managed patient. Obviously, achieving this presents substantial logistical problems when large numbers of individuals are involved and large numbers of tests, procedures, and information-gathering instruments are available for inclusion or exclusion at any one assessment. The computer becomes an essential tool for the Level II manager to be able to schedule and construct this varying type of data update. In fact, although the full potential is still in the future, it is possible that the computer (acting on information fed in by Level III management) might increasingly be able to substitute for the Level II manager in deciding what are appropriate examination compositions and frequencies for individual patients.

When a lifetime health strategy for a patient has been initiated, the Level II manager must almost immediately begin the process of evaluating its results. To do this, information must be obtained to show where the plan is achieving its objectives and where alternative methods need to be tried. This involves one of the most essential but most troublesome concepts in HCM—the concept of a unit of management. In any system that is being managed, some dissection of the system into its component parts is necessary in order for the functional relationships within the system to be comprehended. Similarly, any management plan is itself composed of conceptual if not actual piece parts. It is these piece parts or units of management that we have labeled monads.

At Level I, a monad will ordinarily be the management of an individual episode of illness or injury. The manager will visualize the monad as a divergence or deterioration from the usual norm for the patient and the implicit management objective for the monad will be to return the patient to his norm in the shortest possible time at an acceptable cost. The monad begins with the identification of the divergence and the initiation of management. It ends when the norm is restored or when a stable state is reached with no realistic prospect for further progress. Monads may be counted, measured, evaluated, and otherwise manipulated as needed to assist in quantifying the management process and in measuring progress toward the objective of better health.

Identification of individual monads at Level II is equally desirable and no less useful than at Level I, but considerably more difficult for a variety of reasons. In the first place, Level I monads resemble somewhat the disease entities and nomenclature with which the physician is already familiar, making both the identification of the monad and selection of a suitable name by which to refer to it a reasonably simple process. On the other hand, such preexisting identities are not ordinarily found at Level II, making it harder to conceptualize the monad, and a ready title or name is not always available to serve as its descriptor. Then, with the exception of those physicians who are specially trained or experienced in preventive and constructive medical concepts, Level II presents an unfamiliar and therefore potentially insecure area of activity. In addition to this, the whole arena in which Level II management operates and the state of the art of its various component bodies of knowledge (preventive medicine, prospective medicine, constructive medicine, predictive medicine, wellness medicine, and so on) are in their infancy (though rapidly evolving). Hence, there is little foundation or experience to provide the Level II manager with ready-made monad identities.

It is understandable, therefore, that the monad concept is somewhat difficult for the physician who normally does not regard what he does for the patient as a management function. Furthermore, in the usual physician-patient relationship today the physician is actually not the manager. The *patient* is. The physician only provides certain services that the patient serving as his own manager perceives as being necessary at that particular time.

Consequently, it is difficult for a physician involved for the first time with HCM to grasp the significant difference between what he has always done for a patient and that represented by the term "management of the patient's health." Yet, the physician (and to a limited extent the nurse) must become a manager of health at Level I and at Level II if HCM is to work. This means a significant adjustment. It requires accepting considerably broader objectives than diagnosis and treatment of the presenting condition. It requires acceptance of the challenge to manage all aspects of the patient's health, not just the immediate medical aspects. It requires taking the initiative to stimulate the patient to do what is best for his own health. And it requires coordination and assessment of the real worth of the whole process.

Unfortunately, that feeling of familiarity that the typical physician finds in Level I management is the cause of the two most serious problems associated with physicians' early performance as part of HCM. First, the physician who had been in clinical practice, seeing much in Level I that resembles his former practice of diagnosis and treatment of episodic illness, says to himself, "Why, Level I management is the same thing that I've been doing all along except it's dressed up with a new name. It's really nothing more than just good medical practice." Having concluded this, he relaxes with the conviction that he "can continue to do what he has always done." The truth of the matter is, however, that Level I management requires more than just good medical practice and the physician who does not recognize this cannot be very effective as a part of HCM at Level I.

In much the same fashion, the occupational physician when first faced with HCM is apt to conclude that Level I management is the same as the health counseling with which he is familiar. Unfortunately, this is not the case either, and the occupational physician finds that he has to considerably broaden and extend his concepts to embrace the full implications of Level I management.

The second unfortunate effect of the physician's seeming natural familiarity with Level I management is that Level I will get all his attention and Level II will be neglected. This will result in an HCM offering to the employee that is little more than simple primary care and will, of course, fail on many counts to attain the full potential of HCM. Unless fully counteracted, these two tendencies on the part of physicians new to HCM are likely to result in a version of HCM preoccupied with delivery of medical care and grossly deficient with respect to most of the ojbectives of the HCM idea: in a nutshell, a costly yet still inadequate program.

When the physician does grasp the full significance of his Level I management opportunities, his first attention is directed to the employee-patient who has been or is in the process of being captured. In other words, the employee seems willing to participate and the relationship with him is maturing nicely. In the course of fostering this relationship the employee will be encouraged to report the development of any symptoms or suspicion of disease that may occur, and to the extent that he is comfortable with the relationship the employee is likely to do this at an earlier time than he would have were he not. There are also two other factors in the industrial environment that serendipitously contribute to earlier utilization by the employee of proferred medical service: the convenient availability of the medical facilities (nearby and easily accessible), and the fact that he (the employee) can get out of work to go to the medical department. This latter is, of course, a two-edged sword that needs to be carefully watched lest the privilege be abused, but the Level I manager can also take advantage of the encouragement it gives to employees to come in early with legitimate complaints.

The Level I manager should therefore be hearing sooner or later from each participating employee who will make contact regarding symptoms or will have some health question The latter of course can be satisfied by providing the necessary information. If however, symptoms or suspicions of disease are the instigators of contact, the manager's problem is to make a judgment (perhaps tentative) as to the significance of the presenting symptoms. If they appear to be of little significance, the employee can be reassured. At this point, the manager will also take the opportunity to reaffirm his desire for the employee to report all symptoms even though they turn out to be of no consequence. Thus, the employee is reassured both as to his health and as to the legitimacy of his use of the new relationship with his medical manager.

When significant symptoms are presented, the Level I manager will naturally take whatever steps are necessary to reach a definitive diagnosis and undertake therapy to resolve the problem. An important decision which the Level I manager makes at this point is where to obtain the needed diagnosis and treatment. Should he provide one or both in-house or procure one or both from community resources? There is no one right answer to this question for all situations. The manager must take into account many factors and act accordingly.

The most important factor bearing on this decision is, of course, the quality and competence of available sources of care. The manager will want to use the best available. Also important is the extent to which the employee already has a working relationship with a physician in the community who may be able to provide the medical services. Another consideration, which has been mentioned before, is that the manager needs to deliver a certain amount of diagnostic and therapeutic "laying on of hands" himself in order to help capture and hold the patient in a mutually satisfying relationship. Patients will vary greatly with respect to the amount of such personal medical care delivery they require to give them the confidence in their manager that they need. Some will be perfectly happy with a manager who only manages and advises, with little or no clinical reinforcement. Others will not feel comfortable relating to anyone who does not measure up to thier image of "my doctor." This means, of course, that they expect clinical care personally provided by the doctor. However, even the most demanding patient does not expect "his doctor" to do everything. He will accept referral to specialists, for surgery, and for services clearly outside the field of his doctor without in any way diminishing his confidence in his doctor.

What the Level I manager seeks to do, therefore, is to personally provide enough clinical care to maintain the patient's confidence but resist the temptation to provide all the services he feels competent to perform. If he succumbs to this temptation, he can become so involved with clinical care delivery (which he could have procured from competent sources elsewhere) that he has no time left for those HCM functions that cannot be obtained elsewhere. As a result the HCM program will again have been reduced to little more than simple primary care delivery.

Most commonly, the Level I manager will decide to go to the community for the needed diagnostic or therapeutic services or both and he will ordinarily select an appropriate community physician. If the patient already has a strong relationship with some physician (whom he may refer to as his "personal physician" or "family doctor"), the Level I manager will lean heavily toward selection of that physician rather than some other. On the other hand, the patient may have no personal physician or have a personal physician in name only and no substantive relationship between the two actually exists. In that case, the manager will be freer to select a community physician based on his qualifications for the problem at hand. The patient may, however, have some ideas of his own as to whom to select. If so, the manager will be well advised to give significant weight to the patient's desires.

It should be noted that the manager (with varying amount of input from the patient) selects or procures the services of a community physician. The patient is not "referred" to the community physician. This is an important distinction that sets HCM apart from traditional practice in occupational medicine. In the latter, employee-patients are literally referred to "their own doctor" or having no doctor they are assisted in locating a doctor to whom they can be "referred." The important point is that not only the patient but also the responsibility for that patient is transferred (referred) from the occupational physician to the patient's doctor. As a matter of fact, typically after referral, the occupational physician feels no further responsibility and makes no further attempt to follow the patient's progress. Indeed, he probably will not have any further contact with the patient unless and until the patient himself initiates an additional contact. By contrast, it is an essential concept of HCM that the manager has committed himself to look after the patient and that includes maintaining that posture right on through and beyond an episode where outside help is called in to deal with a particular problem. Thus, the patient is not referred to a community physician and forgotten; the community physician is called in to work with the patient and the manager for a common purpose. Obviously, the community physician will have something to say about this and some community physicians will want no part of such an arrangement, preferring to take total responsibility for the patient or none at all. It may not be possible for the manager to effectively utilize such a physician, although this conclusion should not be reached prematurely. In many cases where the community physician may at first react negatively to the idea of a shared patient, he later finds this no different than what he has always done when he has been called in consultation or accepted a referred patient from a colleague.

Ideally, of course, procurement of the community physician is done directly by the Level I manager who can then explain the situation exactly and make clear just what is desired and what support the company medical service is prepared to offer. Such an initial contact also prepares the way for ongoing communication between the Level I manager and the community physician— an absolute necessity for achieving maximum yield from this partnership of effort.

However, the Level I manager can make direct contact with the community physician only if one or the other of two situations exist: if the HCM program is prepared to pay the fee of the community physician—in which case the Level I manager is in effect hiring the community physician to do a job; or if the patient is willing to have the Level I manager represent him in making that contact. In the latter case, it is essential that the patient fully understand the arrangement in order to prevent future problems. In reality, if the patient is to pay the fee of the community physician (whether with his own dollars or with company benefit dollars is of no importance), he is the one hiring the community physician. This may not be apparent to the community physician when the Level I manager makes the contact unless the manager makes it clear that he is representing the patient and is not assuming responsibility for the patient's bill.

It is clear that setting up the relationship among patient, Level I manager, and community physician to take care of some current illness while the manager continues to pursue his Level II goals for the patient and perhaps even have an ongoing relationship with a second community physician for another current illness in the same patient is indeed a complex process with limitless variations and subtleties. Successful achievement here obviously requires skills that are acquired and improved with experience. In other words, the Level I manager is engaged in practicing a new art—the art of the practice of Level I management.

To the extent permitted by circumstances, the objective is to have the community physician willingly cooperate with the Level I manager. This is a departure from the historical attitude of the community physician toward the occupational physician. The latter is frequently looked upon as and often has to perform from the position of a third-party intruder. Bringing about the desired relationship with the community physician requires communication (with finesse) on the part of the Level I manager; the extent to which he is successful will vary depending on many factors, not the least of which is his own skill in the art of Level I management.

The desired relationship between the Level I manager and the community physician should not be visualized as a one-way street. The Level I manager should be prepared to offer support to the community physician that will make the latter's cooperation more attractive and will result in better care for the patient. Following are some of the tangible contributions that can be made to the community physician:

Information from the patient's baseline record and subsequent recorded findings that may be pertinent

Free laboratory tests (performed by the medical department's laboratory)

Free x-rays taken in the medical department

Free electrocardiograms taken in the medical department

Other tests or procedures that may be available in the medical department

Monitoring of certain parameters at intervals over a period of time, for example, checking the patient's blood pressure at weekly intervals, and reporting the results to the community physician

Providing instruction for the patient on a selected subject, for example, instruction of the diabetic in the use of the insulin syringe

Consultation—either by specialists on the medical department staff or by community experts paid by the medical department

In offering support of the above kinds to the community physician, the Level I manager should make it clear that these (and perhaps other) services are available but the community physician is under no obligation to use them if he would prefer to obtain his support services elsewhere. Thus, HCM presents no threat to the community physician but can, if accepted, be viewed as a great help in providing better patient care. For example, one community physician had not succeeded in controlling a patient's hypertension using the common antihypertensive drugs. He had wanted to use another drug that required more frequent checking of the patient's blood pressure response in order to use it safely, but since it was not practical for him to monitor the patient at the required frequency he had stayed with the less effective drugs. When a Level I manager offered him free monitoring of the patient's blood pressure at any interval he prescribed, he immediately switched to the desired drug and the patient's blood pressure was brought to normal.

Given the cooperation of the employee-patient, all the forces associated with HCM tend inexorably toward the production of the ideal relationship among the HCM manager, the community health care providers, and the patient—ideal that is, from the HCM standpoint of providing the opportunities for better quality medical care and better resulting health at controlled costs. However, having provided the opportunity is one thing; taking advantage of that opportunity is another matter. In the final analysis the results achieved depend on the skills of the HCM manager.

Industry's Medical Involvement Today

H. A. Sinclaire

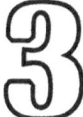

   In the late 1700s Dr. Ramazzini, father of occupational medicine, asked his patients, "Of what trade are you?" He believed that there was frequently a correlation between the patient's morbidity and his work. Now, over 200 years later, how is occupational medicine adjusting to the times? Are physicians still asking about their patients' work history? If they aren't, they should be!

   Directing Mobil Oil Corporation's multiple in-plant health care clinics serves to emphasize that, more than ever before, the medical profession and industry are allied. Civilization has been going through a series of rapid changes from the agrarian economy to the economy based on privately owned and operated enterprises where most people work for the "company" or for some other person who is the "boss." Specialization and other mass production techniques have thrown large groups of people together in their work to a point where it is increasingly difficult for the individual to see himself in relation to the problems and objectives of the business enterprise. This causes tensions and other health problems that are becoming increasingly important in our business life.

As today's industrial civilization has developed, business management as well as other parts of our community have been too slow in adapting to changing conditions. As our work force is brought together in larger and larger groups, many of us are inclined to believe that all problems can be best handled on a group basis. Many of these problems can be so handled without encroaching on the rights of individuals, but there are also many that can still be best handled on an individual basis. One of these is proper attention to the personal health problems of the employee.

The youth of the restless 1960s has grown up and moved into the work force. They expect and demand to be healthy workers with a satisfactory life style. Thus, physicians practicing occupational medicine are committed to protecting and improving the health of workers, thereby contributing to the profit side of the ledger.

During the past forty years there has been a phenomenal increase in the amount of insurance benefits paid to cover employees' sickness and disability. The actual and potential costs of these insurance programs are frightening to many American businessmen. Because these costs affect company profits, the concern of the average businessman responsible for the financial success of his company is understandable. Not only is he alarmed at rising costs caused by increased contributions negotiated at the bargaining table, but he is concerned at the astounding increase in the cost of medical care. National expenditures for health care grew 13 percent from $104.2 billion in 1974 to $117.6 billion in 1975. Today, the average company pays part or all of the premiums for major medical insurance, accident and sickness benefits, and certain life insurance policies. The cost of these benefits must be added to the high cost of doing business.

Many businessmen have accepted these added costs as an inevitable burden of running a business. Managers and physicians frequently ask, "Does an occupational health program pay its way?" Or, "Can you demonstrate a financial return from such a program?" Some resign themselves by replying, "You can't put a price tag on health." Or, "Health has intrinsic values that are not subject to arithmetic calculations." Like it or not, industry in the 1970s is committed to operating comprehensive occupational health programs for its employees. Everything possible must be done to prevent or detect health problems that affect employees and their productivity.

Costly though an industrial health program may be, its alternative is more expensive. When a worker is sick, he is obviously not as productive as he is when he is well. If he is absent because of illness, production is affected. Besides, his salary has to be paid for a time. If the employee does not have the security of a medical insurance program, psychological or morale problems can be created. There are many intangible costs that cannot be measured by industy in having in-plant health care clinics, but it is firmly believed that having a preventive medical program is less costly than not having one.

Today, broad aspects of occupational medicine are influenced by federal regulations, new medical technology, and the work force itself. The 1970s have brought more government involvement to American businesses than ever before. New federal regulations are having and will continue to have an impact on industry's health services. Of particular importance are the Occupational Safety and Health Act of 1970, the Health Maintenance Act of 1973, and the Toxic Substances Control Act of 1976.

Government's Impact on Occupational Medicine

The Occupational Safety and Health Act (OSHAct) was passed in December 1970 and became effective in April 1971. This law is concerned with making the workplace safe and healthy for the employed. Employers are now responsible for ensuring that the environment in which their employees work meets prescribed standards for safety and health. The law, administered by the Department of Labor, stipulates that government inspectors audit the workplace and levy fines when violations are found.

The act has ramifications for occupational medicine in terms of standards, physical examinations, industrial hygiene surveys, new plant construction, and medical support services. The National Institute of Occupational Safety and Health (NIOSH), a branch of the Department of Health, Education, and Welfare, is charged with recommending the standards of health applicable to the workplace. To date, health standards have been proposed by NIOSH which may become regulations enforced by OSHA for controlling or limiting employee exposure to the following: ammonia, arsenic, asbestos,* benzene, carbon monoxide, cotton dust, carcinogens,* heat, hydrogen sulfide, ketones, lead, silica, sulfuric acid, vinyl chloride,* and noise. Because standards are being prepared for hundreds of additional substances, this part of the medical program will continue to expand.

The law also requires industry to give more physical examinations than in the past. Although periodic examinations have always been mandatory for some Mobil Oil Corporation employees, such as pilots and workers exposed to radiation, Mobil now incurs the cost of providing mandatory examinations for 3,380 employees annually, versus 1,320 in 1965, in order to ensure compliance with OSHA standards. Not only have costs risen because of more examinations, but the costs of individual examinations have increased (with laboratory costs more than doubled in the past five years).

To assure that safe and healthy working conditions are being achieved and maintained under the act, industrial hygiene surveys must be performed. Based on these surveys, recommendations are made for correcting conditions that could otherwise result in citations and fines by OSHA inspectors. With the advent of OSHAct, it has become increasingly appreciated that savings can be made by using the precepts of industrial hygiene in the initial design phase of new plant and equipment. To redesign after construction is expensive. Mobil Oil Corporation has recently spent about $400,000 to redesign one refinery to meet the OSHA noise standard, about $250,000 to have a second conform to the

*FDA regulation in the *Federal Register.*

hydrogen sulfide standard, and several thousand dollars to have another plant's ventilation meet the air quality standard.

OSHA's many requirements have increased support services to the health program, thus incurring additional costs. Additional clerical time is needed for maintaining prescribed records. Computer time and data processing services are necessary to perform analyses and prepare reports required not only by government regulations but by union agreements. Extra training time is needed to ensure official certification of technicians. Thus it is clear that OSHA has resulted not only in an increased medical program budget but in many additional costs to industry.

A second time in the 1970s Congress passed a health law affecting industry. A health maintenance organization (HMO) is usually a group practice organization, resembling the Kaiser-Permanente organization, which provides comprehensive health care services on a prepaid basis to its members. Since 1973, the Health Maintenance Act has mandated that if a federally qualified HMO is available, an employer must allow his employees to belong to it if they so wish. No company may force employees to accept company medical plans. Also, employees who join an HMO must be provided with the same financial support they would receive for other medical coverage. If HMOs become an important feature of medical life in this country, we will have to assess how best we can coordinate our medical programs with them.

Congress passed the Toxic Substances Control Act late in 1976. The intent of this legislation is to supplement such existing laws as OSHAct and the various FDA and EPA regulations; it requires premarket notification to the EPA of all new chemical substances at least ninety days before manufacture. For chemical products already on the market, the EPA administrator can require biological testing, labeling, or, indeed, any restriction judged necessary to prevent an environmental hazard.

A multiplier effect is seen in the impacts of legislation on costs to business. At a time when the cost of individual product testing is increasing, a larger number of product tests and more in-house toxicological expertise can be anticipated. The toxicity of each industrial material or product as it relates to a worker's exposure in the process of manufacture as well as to a purchaser's in the course of use will have to be reported on. The evaluation of the toxic properties will have to include studies to determine whether the material can cause cancer, mutations of genes, or deformities of the fetus in early pregnancy; the latter information is increasingly pertinent as more women assume "blue-collar" employment.

It is not possible at this time to assess the full impact of this legislation. It seems certain, however, that hundreds of chemicals and products, both new and already in use, will have to be tested. The Toxic Substance Control Act may lead industry to conclude, in some cases, that the risk of manufacturing a product and the cost of the testing and the protective devices required will not be offset by the return in the marketplace. Thus, a product may be dropped from the list of products manufactured and marketed, adding to the economic effects of this legislation.

Impact of New Technology on Occupational Medicine

In the past ten years there have been developments in medical practice and medical technology that have affected our occupational health programs. Automated laboratory tests and advanced techniques for evaluating the electrical activity of the heart (stress electrocardiography) are examples of new ways that permit earlier detection of disease conditions and, usually, more effective treatment. The result has been an increase in the number and complexity of tests included in the periodic physical examination. In the area of diagnosis and treatment there have also been changes. The application of technology has expanded traditional services so that now, for example, many health care clinics have defibrillators and monitoring devices for treatment of on-the-job cardiac emergencies.

Also in recent years, the "boundaries" of occupational medical practice and company medical programs have become less rigid so that additional services are offered. As a result, many nonoccupational chronic conditions, such as hypertension and diabetes, are being treated in industrial medical facilities. This benefits employees who might not otherwise receive treatment because they find that private physicians are unavilable or are uninterested in these conditions. This benefits industry in the short run since time lost from work for medical care is minimized. The employee and the company benefit in the long run since treatment of hypertension, for example, reduces the risk of heart attack and stroke and prolongs life.

Impact of Today's Work Force on Occupational Medicine

Our work force in the 1970s calls for additional types of medical care because workers are older, because workers include the handicapped, and because workers are subject to a variety of medical conditions brought about by stress. The "average" Mobil Oil Corporation employee of today is older than ten years ago: of 31,000 employees 55 percent are over forty. These older, more experienced workers represent an important company asset. Medically, however, older personnel run an increased risk of illness and death from heart disease, cancer, and other causes. It is estimated that an employee over forty who is overweight, has high blood pressure, smokes, and has an elevated cholesterol level is ten times more likely to have a heart attack than one who has controlled these risk factors.

In addition, a growing number of employees with handicaps and disabilities have joined our work force. In the past, industry's hiring of the handicapped was voluntary. Today, it must be done to comply with federal regulations. These workers necessarily have medical restrictions on their duties in their present assignments and often have limited opportunities for advancement or transfer. In addition, in many but by no means all cases, their health problems can reduce their working lives as well as their overall life expectancy. Medically, we can help minimize these problems by assuring complete understanding of them when the individual is hired and careful reassessment at the time of the periodic examinations.

Mental health is a major element of the overall health of the work force. Changes have occurred here also which are basically the result of increased employee exposure to stress. This stress has several origins: management decisions involving reorganizations, objectives, measures of performance, and job security; the mployee's loss of job flexibility because of aging, acquisition of desirable benefits, and limited alternatives; and strain on family and other social relationships caused by employee transfers, relocations, the "energy crisis," and so on. Such stress produces anxiety, tension states, and depression. These unhealthy mental states lead to loss of job satisfaction, poor performance, alcohol abuse, and other problems which, in turn, result in further deterioration of mental health. They also result in medical problems such as hypertension and peptic ulcer. In the years 1973–1975, our Mobil clinics recorded the instances of ulcers, anxiety, and hypertension displayed in table 1. Cases of hypertension increased from 192 in 1973 to 747 in 1975. In large part, this increase in reported cases resulted from a concentrated effort to find the hypertensive employees and give them medical treatment. It is believed that many medical problems associated with stress can be minimized through early detection, counseling, and other support.

The National Council on Alcoholism has estimated that approximately 5 percent of the nation's work force are alcoholics. There is no reason to believe that this prevalence rate is any different among Mobil employees whether they work at New York headquarters or elsewhere. Hard drug usage, on the other hand, has not been a significant problem among Mobil's New York employees. However, the indiscriminate use of prescribed medications, such as tranquilizers and sedatives, is more likely to exist in the workplace. Although prevalence rates are not available for drug abuse, it is generally believed that alcoholism among employees is by far the greater of these health problems and, of course, often the result of stress.

Mobil's Occupational Health Programs

Although industrial physicians were hired by Mobil Oil Corporation as early as 1912, the company did not formalize its medical policy until 1952. Twenty-five years later, its basic objectives in serving the company and its employees remain the following:

Selecting employees whose mental and physical conditions meet job requirements;

Maintaining a high level of employee health and physical fitness;

Placing employees in positions for which they are fitted;

Table 1.
Cases of Stress-Related Illness, 1973–1975.

Site	1973			1974			1975[a]		
	Ulcer	Anxiety	Hypertension	Ulcer	Anxiety	Hypertension	Ulcer	Anxiety	Hypertension
Plant A	1	6	0	1	6	24	2	6	47
Office B	2	2	6	2	3	37	6	12	94
Office C	3	26	92	9	35	158	8	35	288
Plant D		3	13	1	3	14		9	20
Plant E		1	15		2	22	2	2	47
TOTAL: All Units	12	65	192	24	69	384	30	102	747

[a]Based on 9 months' experience.

Striving for better observance by employees of the principles of health conservation and improvement; and

Maintaining healthful working conditions.

To achieve these objectives, specific items of the occupational health program are: physical examination, primary health services, follow-up services, and special activities. The examination program includes preplacement physical exams, periodic physical exams, special exams for toxic exposure, legally required exams (pilots, interstate drivers), and return-to-work exams after illness. Primary health services include full coverage for occupational illnesses and injuries and limited coverage for nonoccupational illnesses and injuries. Follow-up services are also provided for chronic diseases. Special activities under the occupational health program include employee counseling, a fitness exercise program, an alcohol and drug abuse program, psychiatric screening, preventive immunizations, cancer detection tests, and health education. Other health-related activities are toxicology analysis of products, environmental hygiene surveys of workplaces, and maintenance of medical records. Exhibit 1 shows the increased functions of Mobil Oil Corporation's health program over a ten-year span.

Most recently, Mobil Oil Corporation has been confronted by the realities of adjusting to all the aforementioned concerns of industry's involvement in medicine today. The need to create a computer bank of toxicological data on some 30,000 Mobil products as soon as possible is almost overwhelming. Equally important is the necessity to produce a medical surveillance system to track an employee's work history, hazardous exposure, and medical tests during his entire career. This challenges even the computer's skill, not to mention the intellect of the programmer. Toxicology data, results of industrial hygiene surveys, and employees' work assignments must all be computerized to permit quick retrieval of related information when there is a threat to a worker's health.

Industry's medical records are taking on new dimensions of importance as medical research correlating employee health to work exposure is demanded by the employees, their unions, and the federal government alike. Maintaining the time-honored tradition of patient confidentiality is causing many industrial medical clinics to keep two sets of employee health records—one accessible only to the medical personnel, the second for the OSHA inspector auditing the results of mandatory medical tests such as hearing measurements and asbestos exposures.

Other Corporations' Health Activities

The occupational physician recognizes the primary benefit of the occupational health program to the employee. In turn the employee will feel reassured when he gets high quality health services promptly and pleasantly when it is

Exhibit 1
Ten-year Summary of Increasing Scope of Mobil Medical Services and Functions

	1965	1970	1975
Periodic Exams	Physical exam Chest x-ray Simple blood count Serology Urinalysis Vision test Standard EKG Resting Pap smear Consultations	Added: 10 Chemical tests on blood Hearing measurement EKG on computer Proctosigmoidoscopy	Added: 26 tests on blood EKG with stress exercise
Diagnosis and Treatment	Treatment of occupational injury and illness Emergency care of nonoccupational injury and illness	Added: Some routine care of minor nonoccupational injury and illness	Added: Routine care of major nonoccupational injury and illness (hypertension, adult-onset diabetes. etc.)
Mandatory Surveillance Exams	Drivers Pilots Lead Radiation	Added: Benzene	Added: Asbestos Cholinesterase Organic Phosphate Elemental phosphorus Silica
Environmental Health Functions	Industrial hygiene service upon request	Initiation of regular industrial hygiene surveys in plants employing more than 50	Routine industrial hygiene surveys Courses in constant monitoring for safety and technical personnel, and supervision of same Toxicology of products Product labeling

the responsibility and advantage of the employer to provide it. At the same time the physician wonders how the program under his direction compares with other occupational health services. For that reason B.F. Goodrich Company's recent survey was a welcome opportunity to compare Mobil's health services with those of the participating organizations. B. F. Goodrich surveyed eighty companies in early 1975. Chemical, metal, transportation, petroleum, rubber, and plastics organizations with 5,000 to over 100,000 employees took part in the review. The results provide a basis for evaluating the current relative position of Mobil's medical program.

The various companies employed zero to one full-time physician per 2,000 employees. Mobil has one full-time physician per 2,000 employees in domestic operations. The domestic nursing staff in Mobil is one for every 1,500 employees in comparison with the other companies which reported zero to two nurses for every 1,500 employees. Mobil clinics are equipped as well as or better than many of the eighty companies in the study. Only about half the companies responding had cardiac resuscitation equipment, whereas the majority of Mobil's clinics have such equipment. Mobil's capabilities include clinical laboratory services, x-ray, physiotherapy, and vision, hearing, and heart testing equipment for examination and diagnosis of employees' physical status. Of the companies in the B.F. Goodrich study, 93 percent reported

Exhibit 2
Multicompany Comparison of Medical Services

Services Offered	% of Companies Offering Service	Status of Mobil's Service
Preplacement Physical Exam	96%	Mandatory-100%
Periodic Physical Exam for all Employees	None	Voluntary (78% acceptance)
Environmental Health Exam	75%	Mandatory-100%
Promotion Exam	33%	Voluntary
Overseas Exam	77%	Mandatory
Management Physical Exam	82%	Voluntary (Mandatory for those participating in Fitness Program)
Medical Counseling by Professional Staff	82%	Available in all clinics
Treatment of Occupational Conditions	91%	Available in all clinics
Limited Treatment of Nonoccupational Conditions	87%	Available in all clinics
Physical Conditioning for Management	26%	Available at headquarters on a pilot study

having vision and hearing testing equipment and three-quarters reported having electrocardiograph capabilities. Additional comparisons resulting from the survey are presented in exhibit 2.

Keeping pace with medical technology, government regulations on industrial health, and still remaining true to the employee-patient makes adjusting to the requirements of 1977 a monumental task for the physician in industry.

Union Health Clinics

Thomas Herriman

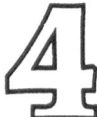

When unions act as direct providers of health care they can have a dramatic impact on the cost and quality of the care their members receive. However, fewer unions operate health centers than ever before, and the number is probably still declining. Among those union sponsored efforts remaining, three bear closer examination: two clinics operated by the Amalgamated Clothing and Textile Workers (ACTWU) in St. Louis and Chicago, and some programs conducted by the United Mine Workers (UMW).

The philosophy behind the ACTWU clinics and the efforts of other unions has been something like: "Our members are entitled to the best medical care that is available, yet they aren't getting it." The ACTWU and several major industrial unions have traditionally seen the union's role as reaching beyond the shop floor and encompassing more than the issues in a union contract. The ACTWU believed, and still does, that almost anything that can be done to improve the lives of its members both at work and off the job would be a legitimate area for union activity.

As a result, the ACTWU pioneered in the establishment of low-cost cooperative housing for working families, established scholarship and educa-tion-by-right programs for children, operates day care centers in Baltimore and Chicago serving several thousand families, operates retiree centers, includes social service workers on its staff, and of course operates health centers.

Today the ACTWU has health centers in New York, Rochester, Baltimore, Philadelphia and Allentown, Pennsylvania, and in Chicago. They serve over 100,000 active members, families, and retired members. The centers were established to meet a need: financial barriers and other problems had prevented people from getting the medical care they needed. Working families rarely received preventive medicine or the health education that goes along with it. Through establishing the centers, the unions hoped to provide more and better health care to their members at a lower cost than would otherwise be possible. In many cases they succeeded very well.

To put the ACTWU activities in perspective, it is important to keep in mind that most unions do not operate health centers. They merely act as purchasers of health insurance, and their members arrange individually for physician and hospital care.

As purchasers of group insurance for union members, unions have vir-tually no impact on the quality or cost of medical services that their members receive. It is only when unions become direct providers that they begin to have some control over these items.

The UMW Appalachia Program

One of the most extensive union health programs is the one conducted by the United Mine Workers. In the 1950s the UMW program included the construction and operation of ten hospitals in the coal fields in Appalachia. These were established in areas where the miners and their families had no other source of hospital care. In the 1960s when union membership in those areas declined, the union sold the hospitals, and they are now operated by a private church-affiliated group. When the union owned them, almost all the patients in the hospitals were miners and the hospital bills of the miners and their families were completely paid by the UMW Welfare and Retirement Fund, which is made up of royalty payments based on each ton of coal that is mined. The hospitals were also open to community members, who had to make their own financial arrangements. Today, about half the income of the hospitals and half the patients come from the communities rather than the miners.

Even though the hospitals have been sold, the union still conducts a vigorous program to monitor the health care received by the 800,000 miners, miners' family members, and retirees covered by the fund. They have instituted several programs to control costs and upgrade quality where their members live. A major thrust is the sponsorship or encouragement of community-based HMO-type clinics in mining areas.

The UMW Welfare and Retirement Fund which pays for the medical programs operates on the assumption that cost control is inherent in all quality control, and that by improving quality one automatically helps to control the cost of medical care. This was stated by Dr. Loren Kerr who formerly served as assistant to the executive medical officer of the fund. For example, the fund pays for surgery only when performed by a board-certified physician. The rate of hospitalization for surgery dropped by 60 percent when the policy was first adopted in the early 1950s. Later, it remained at a level 50 percent below the previous experience, according to Dr. Kerr.

The UMW stimulated the formation of several clinics on the principles of nonprofit operation, consumer sponsorship, prepayment, comprehensive services with an emphasis on prevention, and salaried physicians in a group practice setting. In Madisonville, Kentucky, to take just one example, the UMW worked out an arrangement with the Trover Clinic operated by the Clinic Health Care Plan. When the practice of capitation payments was introduced in paying for health services to the beneficiary population, it was found that hospital utilization and costs decreased by 30 percent and 25 percent respectively over a two-year period.[1]

The UMW is also experimenting with the "managing physician concept," a unified approach to personal health care embodying the best features of the traditional family doctor combined with ready access and referral to a wide range of specialized services. Use of the concept has permitted substantial reductions in hospital days in some pilot programs. In many areas. the union has encountered substantial opposition to establishing clinics on this basis. They were fought bitterly by the medical societies in the Bellaire area, although the dust seems to have settled and the clinic is accepted by the rest of the medical community.

It is important to note that it was the union that took the initiative in calling for departures from the traditional practice of medicine. It is the union that is the innovator in this and many other cases, an important role that few other groups or institutions are able or willing to serve. Unions do not have a vested interest as part of the medical establishment; they have a strong interest in saving money, since negotiated funds necessary to pay health benefits reduce the amount that can be negotiated in wage increases; and they have a sincere and idealistic interest in the general health and well-being of their members. Unfortunately, unions that want to operate their own centers face some obstacles that may be insurmountable.

The ACTWU Sidney Hillman Health Center

The Sidney Hillman Health Center in Chicago serves several thousand union members and their families who work in the men's clothing industry in the city. It was established in 1962 and for many years was the only union-sponsored health center in the city. The Sidney Hillman Health Center is an HMO-type health provider. The patients are a voluntarily enrolled population of ACTWU members in Chicago who are provided both outpatient and inpatient care for prepaid fixed premiums. The hospital services are covered by the Amalgamated Life and Health Insurance Company. The center provides for the fixed premiums, dental excluding orthodontia, eye, drugs at no cost, laboratory. x-ray. physiotherapy, all physician services primary and secondary, and social services including counseling and referrals. There is a full-time medical director and a staff of forty to fifty physicians who work on a part-time basis.

The employers under contract to the union in the city pay a percentage of gross payroll into the Amalgamated Social Benefits Association which operates the clinic. The Amalgamated Social Benefits Association also provides hospitalization and life insurance for the union members. The combination of the clinic and the insurance program covers virtually 100 percent of the medical costs that union members incur. As a result, most union members have very limited out-of-pocket expenses for medical care.

The insurance company is completely owned and operated by the union. This stems from the fact that in the 1940s when the union sought to purchase group health insurance from private carriers, exhorbitant fees were demanded. Thus, both the insurance company and the clinic were set up because union members needed services that could not be provided elsewhere. In addition, of course, the union knew the economic value of doing things in a group. It made sense to apply the group concept to medical care.

Every union member who is enrolled in the clinic goes through a series of screening tests and an initial physical examination. Since there are no charges for doctor visits, members do not have a financial barrier when they find they have medical questions or problems. The diagnostic program, coupled with the encouragement of regular visits, has resulted in a substantial reduction in the number of days spent in the hospital by members using the center.

The Sidney Hillman Health Center requires a mandatory second opinion prior to medical or surgical hospitalization by any health center physician. In addition, there are quarterly reviews of patient utilization of physician services at the center by the medical director for control of over- or underutilization. In addition, there is a regular review by the medical director of all referrals by internists to orthopedics, neurology, rheumatology, and so forth. In addition to the quality of care review programs, all hospital admissions are monitored very closely. According to ACTWU researcher Jeannette Wilson, the hospitalization rate for Sidney Hillman Health Center members was 390 days per 1,000 patients in 1976. There were 4,748 active patients and 183 admissions totaling 1,852 hospital days. Excluding Medicare, the rate was 292 days per 1,000 patients. The Medicare rate was 678 days per 1,000 patients.

By contrast, the national average for hospitalization for people in prepaid groups was beteen 425 and 450 per 1,000. Co-Care, an HMO facility in Chicago operated by Blue Cross, showed a hospitalization rate of 709 per 1,000. The national average for hospital days per 1,000 people enolled in private insurance plans including Blue Cross was between 799 and 825 per 1,000, according to figures recently compiled by the Committee for National Health Insurance.

Clearly, the union is doing something right. Part of the explanation for the lower hospitalization rates lies in the utilization controls. But another aspect clearly lies in the willingness of people to use the clinic. The Sidney Hillman Health Center is located near some of the large workplaces in Chicago, and has been in operation nearly twenty years. Clearly, the habits people develop in using the clinic, how comfortable they feel there, and how familiar they are with the idea of preventive medicine are important factors in utilization control.

Cost control is extremely important to unions. Any trade unionist who negotiates contracts that include health bnefits must be acutely conscious of the rise in cost of health care. With each contract renewal, more money must be negotiated from the employers just to pay the inflationary price increases for benefits that people already have. To add to benefits, still more money is necessary.

In the ACTWU we are perhaps more acutely aware of the rise in helath costs than in many other industries and unions. In 1974 our entire health insurance program went through a severe crisis that stemmed from the deep recession experienced by the men's clothing industry at that time. Nearly 100,000 people work in the industry, which was hit by extremely high unemployment resulting from a nationwide recession and from high levels of imports. Workers with ten years' seniority in the men's clothing industry may claim health insurance benefits for up to a year after they are laid off. After a worker is laid off, employers no longer contribute funds to the health plan on their behalf. Consequently, a sharp drop in employer contributions occurred while the level of claims remained high and the fund was in a financial crunch. The union members were entitled to receive a $0.325 an hour wage increase in June 1974. Instead of taking the wage increase on their pay checks, they voted overwhelmingly to transfer the money that would have been due them for four months into the health fund to make sure that it kept solvent.

The ACTWU is one of the most politically active unions. It is working for passage of national health insurance, and on the practical level of providing health care of their members, it is vigorously investigating HMO options and a variety of methods of cost control and quality control that will continue to permit union members to receive high quality medical care at a cost they can afford.

Insurance vs. HMO: A Direct Comparison

In St. Louis, Missouri, the benefit program covering a group of 1,100 textile workers provides a unique opportunity for a direct comparison of the effectiveness of the cost and quality controls practiced in an HMO setting. Under the St. Louis Employers and Amalgamated Clothing and Textile Workers Union Benefit Program, workers in covered employment may select either Blue Cross–Blue Shield medical coverage on the one hand, or they may elect to enroll in the program's health center. If they choose Blue Cross–Blue Shield coverage, which is known as Option A, members and families can use a physician of their choice for hospitalization and surgery. The benefits are not as comprehensive as those of Option B, in which all health services originate in the health center.

Option A provides seventy hospital days (thirty days mental), partial payment of ancillary charges, partial coverage for surgery charges ($350 maximum), and major medical coverage for workers at one of the plants. Under Option B virtually all costs are paid, including all medical services provided by the health center as well as 365 days of hospital room and board and 100 percent of ancillary hospital charges. Under Option B, the health center acts as the family doctor. Fees for medical services provided by outside physicians to outpatients who have been referred to them by the health center physicians are paid by the program as are outside diagnostic laboratory fees. The program also pays for hospitalzation and medical treatment for accidents and medical emergencies. The health center requires members and spouses to take a medical screen examination furnished by an outside provider for which they are partially reimbursed. This procedure is a key factor in the practice of preventive medicine, one of the main goals of the program. Medical care is available on demand at the center, and there are emergency room arrangements at two St. Louis hospitals for hours when the center is closed. The center includes a discount pharmacy, a fully equipped and staffed dental facility, and optical and ophthalmological care, in addition to a full range of physicians' services. Virtually the entire cost of operation of the center is paid by employers under the terms of collective bargaining agreements with the union.

For the year ended February 28, 1977, members covered by Option B and using the program health center had a ratio of 216 hospital days per 1,000 members, while Option A coverage, which provided conventional Blue Cross–Blue Shield coverage without the screening and preventive medicine aspects, showed a ratio of 301 hospital days per 1,000 members. Plan administrator Charles Sallee, an ACTWU vice-president, attributes the dramatic difference in the hospitalization rate of the two groups to the screening examinations and subsequent follow-up of detectable problems, as well as regular review of diagnosis calling for surgery and hospitalization. (The St Louis data are not directly comparable with the Chicago data since the St. Louis data do not include information on length of stay or number of admissions. However, the number of hospital days shown for the two St. Louis groups are directly comparable.)

Why would an intelligent person choose Option A under the St. Louis benefit program instead of Option B which provides a wider range of services at no more cost to the member? There appear to be two reasons: One is that families may live a substantial distance from the health center, making it difficult or inconvenient to use the facility. Another reason is that people may be reluctant to try what they consider to be an unorthodox approach to medical care, preferring to rely on a known family physician. The union in St. Louis finds that it must conduct a steady educational program to make people aware of the benefits they are entitled to under Option B of the program. Under plans offered by some other unions, members are charged more if they select an HMO option. In such cases members have been slow to choose the higher cost option. This cannot be a factor in the St. Louis program, however, where the cost to the member is the same.

Factors Affecting Utilization

At both the Sidney Hillman Health Center in Chicago and the ACTWU clinic in St. Louis, many union members do not use the clinic even though they are eligible. Part of the explanation lies in the constant turnover in the work force and unfamiliarity with the facility. Part of the reason may lie in traditional resistance to using a health provider other than the neighborhood family doctor. But undoubtedly the biggest factor is demographic. People are moving out of the central cities where the clinics are located. Unions are financially hard pressed in keeping the doors open on one clinic, much less opening satellite clinics. If it is not convenient or easy for people to drop into the clinic before or after work or on Saturday, they will not come to the clinic. When they are sick, they will seek care. When they are not sick, or only marginally so, they will not go out of their way to see a doctor.

Some of the techniques for cost control that are practiced as a matter of course in union health centers are being adopted elsewhere. Two unions in New York City that do not operate health centers recently experimented with programs providing a second opinion on surgery. The concept was subsequently enacted into law by the New York legislature and became a requirement for all insurance companies doing business in the state.

The two unions are District Council 37 of the American Federation of State, County and Municipal Employees, with 110,000 members, and the Storeworkers Union. A report on these programs was published by the Council on Wage and Price Stability in 1974.[2] The DC 37 second opinion program is voluntary and covers all 110,000 working union members. A free second opinion is available to any member of the Health and Security Plan who wishes it. Dr. Eugene McCarthy, the organizer of both plans, estimates that under the voluntary program the union health fund saved over $2 million on surgery that was called for in a first opinion but not confirmed in a second opinion. There was a 4.4 percent reduction in elective surgery. Under a mandatory second opinion program, which the Storeworkers Union operated, the savings were more than twice as high, and there was a 9.4 percent reduction in elective surgery.

The Future

In many instances, unions have done an outstanding job in operating health centers and establishing other innovative programs to help provide for the health needs of their members. However, there are probably fewer union health centers in operation today than in 1969, when the Department of Health, Education, and Welfare counted 101 centers serving 1.6 million members,[3] and it is unlikely that many new union clinics will be established in the future. Large, rapid increases in the cost of medical facilities construction makes starting up new centers more difficult. In addition, the high mobility and wide geographic distribution of workers even in a single plant makes the establishment of just one physical facility impractical; utilization would be too low. In the city of Chicago, for instance, it is not uncommon for people who work in the same plant to live 75 or 100 miles apart and 50 miles from the central city. In such a setting it might require five or six locations to adequately serve the majority of the membership.

It is probably only through partnership with other unions and other groups in the community that unions will be able to play a continuing role as direct providers. This is what the UMW has attempted in the coal fields. Several unions including the ACTWU are conducting feasibility studies to see if HMOs can be established that would draw on a wider community than just union membership for an enrollment base.

The AFL-CIO has said that "The best buy for their health care dollar that unions can negotiate for their members is in prepaid group practice plans. Traditional health insurance plans and fee-for-service practice do not provide the quality care that members of good HMOs receive." The real answer to the health care needs of working families lies in enactment of comprehensive national health insurance along the lines of the Kennedy-Corman bill, and along the lines of the Canadian government-operated system. National health insurance continues to be one of the top two or three legislative goals of the American labor movement. Until such time as it is enacted, unions can be expected to continue to experiment with HMO arrangements and other innovative programs that will serve the health needs of their membership.

NOTES

1. Rural Health Care Delivery, Proceedings of a national conference on Rural Health Maintenance Organizations, Louisville, Kentucky, July 8–10, 1974, conducted by the Group Health Association of America, Inc. Prepared for the Subcommittee on Rural Development of the Committee on Agriculture and Forestry, United States Senate (Washington, D.C.: USGPO, 1974), p. 83.

2. The Complex Puzzle of Rising Health Care Costs, President's Council on Wage and Price Stability (Washington, D.C.: USGPO, 1976), pp. 105–113.

3. Health Insurance Plans Other Than Blue Cross or Blue Shield Plans or Insurance Companies, U.S. Department of Health, Education, and Welfare, Social Security Administration, Office of Research and Statistics, Research Report no. 35 (Washington, D.C.: USGPO, 1971), p. 11.

Comprehensive Care through Physicians Serving in Both Corporate and Private Practice

William E. Greer, Warren Kantrowitz, and Philip S. White

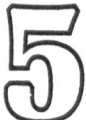

While the debate over what kind of health care system is best for the American people continues, a number of private organizations have long since taken this matter into their own hands. The Gillette Company, a large, diversified, multinational corporation headquartered in Boston, is a notable example of a corporation that maintains its social responsibility to employee and community.

Twenty-five years ago, long before the health care situation became a national issue, The Gillette Company instituted a quality health care program of its own for its employees. This has become a model on which some other socially progressive industrial concerns have developed their programs. The comprehensive Gillette health care program has a range of activities from treating minor industrial injuries to diagnosing and treating acute and chronic illness. It includes preventive medicine through its periodic complete health survey program as well as rehabilitation of cardiac patients, alcoholics, and physically and mentally handicapped employees. In addition to the in-house medical program, the Gillette medical program includes a nurse practitioner who makes hospital and home visits to ill or injured employees to better coordinate and maintain appropriate liaison on current health problems, return to work, and rehabilitation. The health care program carries out a continuous study of occupational stresses and strains. It establishes and maintains health care standards for Gillette divisions throughout the United States and abroad, which include fifty manufacturing facilities in twenty-one countries. While the average American has a valid reason to be concerned about the state of the nation's health care system, a great deal of anxiety has been removed from the Gillette Company employee's search for health care services that are both excellent in quality and abundant in scope.

In contrast to many health care programs, our health care is delivered in a very personalized fashion, with the same physicians caring for employees in the industrial setting and also, in most cases, when they are hospitalized. This allows for a smoother, more efficient system of care, with more opportunities for cost containment. In addition, the program allows for careful, appropriate consultation from specialists without loss of patient control. Should the employee wish to return to a doctor or hospital in his home area, every effort is made by Gillette Medical to cooperate with the local provider. We include free communication of information and ideas on the health problems of the patients, as well as providing reports of follow-up studies performed in our laboratory and x-ray departments.

The staff includes internists, a hematologist, an endocrinologist, surgeons, dermatologists, ophthalmologists, and an allergist. All the physicians also maintain a fee-for-service office practice. The staff are all board-qualified or -certified in their various specialties, and are also medical school faculty members with ongoing teaching responsibilities. In addition to physicians, the staff includes three certified nurse practitioners: one is in charge of the large South Boston facility, another, the Prudential facility, and the third, home and hospital patient liaison.

Since the health of the employee's family is vital to the total health of the employee, many family members are referred by the employees to the private offices of the Gillette staff physicians for medical or surgical care on a fee-for-service basis, utilizing the Blue Cross Master Medical Program. Gillette Boston medical staff maintain close relationships with leading hospitals and specialists in the area. The locally known Gillette philosophy of health care makes for a smooth medical operation and effective delivery of quality care which is often lacking in other health care approaches.

Mental health problems, an increasing challenge, are taken care of by qualified internists where possible, with appropriate referral when indicated but with close contact with consulting psychiatrists in matters of care and rehabilitation. Gillette has an excellent rehabilitation program for persons with alcohol problems, under the capable direction of a rehabilitation and counseling manager. He is a member of the medical team, reporting and responsible only to the medical director. He also is available to provide care to employee family members if they have alcohol problems, and to help them participate in an employee's rehabilitation. Physicians on the Gillette staff are available to employees or their families twenty-four hours daily, seven days a week for outside medical clinic care on a fee-for-service basis.

In most large companies, the concern over the years has been with executive health. The Gillette Company has always taken a broader viewpoint. Gillette management realizes that all men and women employees are important to the industry. Gillette is making increasingly heavy demands on the medical profession for sound guidance concerning matters of employee health maintenance. Safety engineering practice has been developed to a point where most employees are actually safer on the job than at home or on the highway. In-house health programs involve an approach to the total health of the employee by treatment of acute and chronic illness, by periodic health appraisals, by rehabilitative measures, and by health education. Health maintenance involves early detecting of abnormalities and correcting, where possible, the defects. Effectiveness will be demonstrated by reduced sickness, decreased absenteeism, lives saved or prolonged, reduced labor turnover, and improved employee morale.

The comprehensive care approach has the goal of accomplishing the most it can for employee health: preventive, diagnostic, constructive, rehabilitative, and curative medicine are the elements. The rationale of the preventive approach is based on two important considerations: that the earlier a disease is detected, the easier it is to cure or control; and that many illnesses are asymptomatic in the early stages and the average patient does not consult a physician unless he is experiencing symptoms.

The periodic examination of the presumably well individual, or the diagnostic examination of an individual with symptoms not sufficiently severe to cause him to consult a private physician, has real merit. By means of such examinations conducted at no cost to the individual and on company time, many abnormalities are detected in their early stages. This is particularly true of degenerative diseases. Early detection may occur when such conditions are more amenable to either cure or control. Examples of these would include the following which have been detected with some frequency during the course of routine health survey examinations: hypertension, diabetes mellitus, liver disease, arrhythmias and other cardiac conditions, tuberculosis, psychiatric problems, venereal disease, and several common types of cancer. Included in the latter are cancers of the breast, lung, bladder, colon, prostate, blood, skin, mouth, and throat. Many times these diseases are either asymptomatic or the symptoms are so minimal that the employee has not sought medical attention specifically for them. The emphasis should be on preventive medicine—keeping well people well.

It is important to point out, in this era of threats to confidentiality, that the occupational health physician has the same moral, ethical, and legal obligation to his employee-patients as he has to patients in his private practice, and indeed they are often seen as patients in both settings. At The Gillette Company, personal medical records are kept in the medical department and are not subject to review by management. The physician is not controlled by management. Instead, he is present for the benefit of all the employees, from top executives to the lowest paid worker. Although all members of the staff are available to any of the employees, an effort is made to have each employee identify personally with a physician of his choice. This prevents one of the most common objections patients have to care received in a "clinic setting." That is, that they see a different doctor on every visit and not one that really understands or cares for their particular problem.

We would like to emphasize our opinions on the positive value to health of carrying out periodic health surveys, in constrast to the current publicity about health checkups being a "rip-off" by the medical profession. These examinations, an "executive-type" physical survey, are available to all Gillette employees at the industrial clinic and to their dependents on a fee-for-service basis.

The health survey is not designed primarily to make startling discoveries of serious physical impairment, even though defects, both major and minor, will be found. On the average, only about 65 percent of any population seems to have preferred or standard health profiles, meaning that they are free of minor or major defects. The benefits of the health survey are that it:

Preserves good health. This is the primary objective.

Makes people health conscious. It is important to know that you are well. Minor conditions or complaints are often borne in silence as one of the routine burdens inherent in the process of living.

Overcomes fear of examination. Some individuals dread examination because of fears of something seriously wrong being found. If the examination is normal, then considerable apprehension may be relieved.

Banishes false disease symptoms. Some fear disease to such an extent that they may actually experience symptoms of the disease that they secretly believe they have, the most common being heart disease. Dispelling false fears is excellent treatment for getting back into a normal healthy state of mind.

Reveals physical defects. This is not the total motivation for health surveys, but serious problems may be discovered early enough for remedial treatment. Correction or treatment of potentially serious problems discovered may avert later, more serious or chronic conditions or complications.

Reveals causes other than physical defects for poor health such as poor living habits or emotional problems.

Gives an opportunity for teaching good health habits.

There is a close relationship between emotional stress and employee health. The occupational health physician watches for signs of occupational or nonoccupational stress and gives appropriate care. Many employees welcome the opportunity to relieve tensions and stresses and appreciate learning better how to deal with their problems. If stress and its results are due to an unfavorable home situation, the employee can be assisted in understanding the source of the problem. Symptoms such as fatigue may sometimes be due to hard physical effort or advanced disease, but most often are based on a lack of incentive or interest in the job, lack of background for increased responsibilities, imbalance between work and relaxation, lack of physical exercise, or emotional conflict. The treatment may be to direct the patient to a different mode of personal living and thinking. Alteration of style of living has recently become popular as a preventive medicine approach, and some hope it will ultimately reduce health care costs.

The Gillette Medical Department, because of the way the program has developed, deals with a wider range of problems than most physicians on contract for occupational health care. The department is concerned primarily with the health of the work force, and this includes a galaxy of related topics such as personnel, research, absenteeism, safety, compensation problems, composition of health premiums, detection of health hazards, environmental control, retirement decisions, placement of workers in relation to their physical and mental capabilities, community health activities, promotion and reassignment decisions, problems affecting the employment of certain categories of handicapped workers, proper treatment of acute or chronic illness in employees, and counseling on family problems. This can only be accomplished by properly qualified and motivated medical personnel. Of vital importance is knowledge of the health and behavior of individuals as related to their jobs and associates. Based upon the knowledge of employee health and psychology, Medical Department personnel are often involved in evaluation of special company programs and of factors that account for employee morale. It must again be emphasized that the physician–nurse–employee patient relationship is privileged and confidential. The Medical Department also has a significant role in occupational health programs designed to discover, treat, and control a wide range of potential occupational health disorders with a significant morbidity and mortality.

Medical Department visits by Gillette employees in the Boston area for occupational and nonoccupational illnesses and injuries including eye department visits, preplacement, and health survey examinations have been significant in number since its beginning in 1952, averaging about 40,000 visits per year. In 1976, total visits were 45,145. The highest number, 49,046 visits, occurred in 1974. There are approximately 4,500 employees in the Boston area, and the visits to the clinic vary according to the number of employees.
range of potential occupational health disorders with a significant morbidity and mortality.

Medical Department visits by Gillette employees in the Boston area for occupational and nonoccupational illnesses and njuries including eye department visits, preplacement, and health survey examinations have been significant in number since its beginning in 1952, averaging about 40,000 visits per year. In 1976, total visits were 45,145. The highest number, 49,046 visits, occurred in 1974. There are approximately 4,500 employees in the Boston area, and the visits to the clinic vary according to the number of employees.

In addition to the larger South Boston Medical Department, the Gillette Company has recently established a smaller clinic in the Prudential Center for employees in that area. The total employee visits for health reasons to the Gillette Prudential Clinic is about 10,000 per year, with an employee population of 1,600 (thereby increasing the number of visits at the South Boston unit). The South Boston clinic includes an x-ray department, clinical laboratory, eye department, hearing testing, pulmonary function testing, physiotherapy, electrocardiograph, and stress testing. The Corporate Medical Center Clinic in the Prudential Center includes a clinical laboratory, electrocardiograph, and pulmonary function testing. Employees are referred to the South Boston Medical Department for x-ray studies, hearing tests, surgical and dermatological consultations, and eye services. Both clinics are equipped with crash carts and cardiac defibrillation equipment. To date, we have resuscitated four out of six employees who had suffered cardiac arrest at work.

It is important to attempt a crude cost-benefit analysis of these corporate health programs, although they often defy analysis. Realistic goals have to be established if one is to attain effective health cost containment. It is important to try to reduce employee medical expenses by appropriate health programs. Such activities have an obvious impact on health insurance premiums. The Gillette program has attempted to achieve some degree of cost control, without losing sight of the primary objective of providing high quality health care for all Gillette employees.

According to a recent report by Snyder,[1] corporate concern about rising health costs is steadily increasing. Costs for the company's employee health benefit program have risen by 120 percent in six years. The premium increases for Bethelehem Steel have averaged 10 percent annually over the past six years, and premiums now total $115 million. Eastern Airlines has had a 100 percent increase from 1973 to 1976, and now pays $850 per employee annually. Ford Motor Company has been trying to control costs; despite this, company spending for health care rose from $68 million in 1965 to $298 million in 1975. Ford's total expenditures for health care are expected to reach $575 million in 1979.

What has Gillette's recent experience been? Not surprisingly, our health care costs have also been increasing rapidly. In 1970 Gillette had 3,800 employees in the Boston region, and our work force had increased 60 percent by 1976. During this same period, the cost of operating our medical department increased from $330,000 to $710,000 (115 percent). In addition, the cost of purchasing Blue Cross, Blue Shield, and major medical insurance has also increased, despite our greater level of investment in our in-house programs (for example, last year the Medical Department provided laboratory, x-ray, and EKG tests to employees that would have cost $180,000 if obtained from non-Gillette-associated providers). These premium increases reflect an increse of 120 percent since 1972 in the total annual amount paid for claims under these insurance programs ($1.9 million to $4.2 million).

At this juncture, it would be appropriate to quantify the benefits accruing to Gillette and its employees as a result of our in-house programs which offset our rather substantial investment. This is a difficult endeavor and before beginning, we would like to pass on the comment of Dr. Hallett Lewis (director of occupational medicine for the Kaiser Foundation International), who has likened the attempt to measure the cost-benefit effectiveness of an industrial health program to "reaching into a bowl of Jell-O and trying to come up with a handful."[2] Many of the benefits believed to accrue from our efforts do not lend themselves to quantification, and we will mention them only briefly later on. The cost of obtaining the services we provide our employees, and the value of the man-hours that Gillette would forfeit if it could not provide these services at its work sites are, however, easier to estimate.

A detailed study has been made of the visits to, and services provided by, the Gillette Medical Department during 1970. Applying this distribution of services to the known total number of visits made in 1976, as shown in table 1, provides us with an approximation of the services actually provided by the medical department during 1976.

In that year approximately 3,575 special examinations were provided by the Medical Department. If the department had not provided these tests, Gillette would still have had to arrange and pay for the 825 preemployment physical examinations. In addition, approximately 50 percent of the health survey examinations are undertaken at the company's request or policy, and thus represent another company obligation. The remaining health survey and eye examination visits are mostly the result of the voluntary actions of our employees, and we feel that as many as three-quarters of these visits would not be made if the employees did not have convenient access to the Medical Department. Thus, approximately 2,200 of these special examinations would still have been performed if the services had to be acquired by either the company or its employees from outside medical resources. These examinations tend to be among the most comprehensive and expensive services provided by the department, since they involve considerable amounts of ancillary support, and we conservatively estimate that the average cost per examination by outside providers would be $150. The cost (to either the company or its employees) which is therefore saved amounts to $330,000.

Referring again to table 1, we estimate that nearly 8,000 visits were made

Table 1.
Distribution of Visits by Type, 1970 and 1976.

Type of Visit	1970		1976 Total Visits	1976 Estimated Visits by Type
	No. of Visits	% Visits		
Special Exams				
Preemployment	594	1.5		825
Health Surveys	1,497	3.5		1,925
Eye Exams	718	1.5		825
Occupational	6,055	14.5		7,975
Nonoccupational	32,938	79.0		43,450
Total	41,802	100.0	55,000	55,000

to the Medical Department in 1976 for treatment of occupational illnesses and injuries. Naturally, occupational complaints range from the trivial to the critical, and it is quite probable that even if the Gillette in-house resources were considerably more limited than they are, many of the less serious incidents would not be referred to outside sources. Assuming that only 50 percent of these incidents would be referred, and that 80 percent of the referred cases would be sent to private offices (average cost $50) while the other 20 percent would be treated in hospital emergency rooms or outpatient departments (average cost $100), the cost to Gillette for these services would be $240,000.

The largest component of the total visits to the Gillette medical clinics is visits for nonoccupational ailments (43,450 in 1976). As is the case for occupational injuries and illnesses, many of these visits would not have been made except for the convenience and cost advantages to the employee of the medical clinics. Making adjustments for visits for colds, headaches, and other minor complaints, an internal Gillette evaluation of the medical service estimated that 55 to 60 percent of the total nonoccupational visits would be made to outside sources of medical care. In this analysis, we conservatively estimate that only 50 percent of total nonoccupational visits would have actually been made under these circumstances. At an conservatively estimated average cost of $50 per visit (including laboratory, x-ray, and other ancillary services), the cost to Gillette and its employees of obtaining these services from outside sources would have been nearly $1.1 million.

Since the Gillette medical clinics provide an on-site source of medical treatment, employee working time is not lost traveling to, waiting at, and returning from outside medical treatment services. If we assume that all 4,000 visits to outside sources for treatment of occupational illness or injury would have been made during working hours, and that 75 percent of the 21,725 visits for nonoccupational-related medical care, 200 eye examinations, and 1,200 health survey examinations would also have been made during working hours, the total number of visits during 1976 working hours exceeds 21,000. We estimate that two hours of working time, beyond the time spent in providing these services on-site, would have been lost for each of these 21,000 visits. Since the average hourly wage at Gillette is approximately six dollars, the availability of on-site care saved the company another $250,000.

These quantifiable savings total slightly more than $1.9 million for 1976, more than offsetting the $700,000 Medical Department budget. True, there are other costs, such as the time lost from work for convenience visits that otherwise would not be made during working hours (although we strive to minimize these costs), but we feel that these costs are more than offset by the value of the other kinds of benefits accruing to which we cannot, at this time, attach a monetary value. These other "pluses" include:

Control of hospitalization costs since ambulatory studies done by competent physicians avoid excessive hospitalization costs, and the option of instituting second opinion by Gillette physicians on the appropriateness of surgical procedures planned by outside physicians is available in questionable cases.

Gillette's physicians do their own peer review by carefully monitoring one another's records for appropriateness, and can review bills for outside medical services if charges appear excessive or unwarranteed.

Outside referral costs are controlled because specialists on the staff have developed ongoing relationships with their patients.

The health maintenance approach by the Gillette Medical Department emphasizes prevention, early detection, and control of diseases which, we hope, will lead to fewer advanced cases and, consequently, less absenteeism, less staff turnover, and less need to initiate expensive treatment modes.

Personalized services are provided in the Gillette system, and this type of medical care is wanted by our employees (and all patients). If physicians on the staff or associated with the staff of corporate health programs also provide fee-for-service care at their own offices outside the primary clinic facilities, the potential exists for better control of health costs as duplication of charts, work-ups, and laboratory work is eliminated.

The potential total benefits of having physicians participate in both corporate health clinics and fee-for-service office practices are many. The health personnel understand expenses of private practice such as laboratory and x-ray fees, consultation fees, and costs of emergency room care. If physicians participate in both health care programs, there is less institutional near-sightedness and lack of understanding of the "private care" world. In addition, the system can take care of employee families. Serving as primary care physicians for families is good for morale and makes the patient feel that he is not dealing with a company physician, but rather with one who is primarily concerned with the employee and his family's health. There is an understanding of family problems which may lead to work problems. Further, it is possible to control expenses and provide better care of health programs for the employees' families through control of excess hospitalization, the option of an open-panel health maintenance organization, and seven-day, twenty-four hour medical care coverage by physicians.

The physicians also work in hospitals and better understand expenses and can control extra days of hospitalization, extra tests, and extra use of consultants. There is no loss of patient care control. There is an incentive to use less expensive means of patient care such as extended care facilities, visiting nurse specialists, and nurse practitioners for home follow-ups. Physicians who truly understand the health problems of these employee-patients may allow them to return to work earlier than physicians who are not associated with corporate health clinics. Private physicians often have a tendency to be excessively conservative in letting people return to work.

In summary, we have provided an overview of the comprehensive primary health care system which is the Gillette health program, staffed by physicians serving both the corporate health clinic and in fee-for-service office practices. The development of facilities and services designed to accomplish this has resulted in signficant cost savings for both the employee and the company. In addition, the employees are part of a fully integrated and comprehensive corporate-private practice arrangement. More of course needs to be done to plan health care delivery systems by industry to reduce health care costs and simultaneously increase health care coverage for employees and their dependents. We hope that the sharing of our company's experiences with a corporate in-house medical practice that is structurally related to the physicians' fee-for-service office practice will be of interest and importance to others who wish to establish linkages between in-house corporate activity and the private sector of medical practice.

NOTES

1. J. Snyder, "The Fringe Benefit Factor: An End to Business as Usual," *Modern Medicine* 45:17–25, 1977.

2. Hallett A. Lewis, "Determining the Cost Effectiveness of Occupational Health Programs," *Health Care Issues for Industry* (New York: The Conference Board, 1974), p. 30.

A Corporation's Broad-Brush Approach to Meeting Changing Needs

C. Larkin Flanagan, James D. Mortimer, and Richard B. DiBona

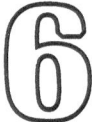

The traditional goal of Continental Bank's Medical Department—the delivery of occupational health care—was intended to minimize fringe benefit costs and provide medical care for employees and customers who were injured or became ill during working hours. The general rule was to hire healthy people and to ensure continuity of medical care insurance coverage if an illness did occur. There was little recognition or corporate commitment to programs that encouraged preventive medical techniques to ensure good health: the medical care system was primarily concerned with crisis invention.

For this purpose, the bank maintained until recently only the following health services.

Preemployment physical examinations to determine eligibility for employment

Drug screening to prevent employment of drug-dependent persons

Emergency procedures to deal with medical crisis situations

Evaluation of employees who returned to work after being out for three days or more

Immunization for employees traveling overseas on business

Physical examinations for employees relocating to overseas assignments

"Sick calls" to employees who become ill or injured while at work

Maintenance of all records required by local, state, and federal laws as related to injury and illness

Screened physician resource list for employees in need of medical attention

Medical consultation about a discovered illness, if requested

Overview of Present and Future Health Benefits

In 1974 a review of various legal, social, and cost factors effected a major shift in our medical care orientation. We discovered that the expectations of our employees coupled with those of society in general were such that a simplistic occupational health program was no longer sufficient. In addition, fringe benefit costs were becoming a significant budgetary item and it appeared that they would increase further unless a more positive approach was initiated.

We therefore shifted our emphasis to an occupational medical counseling/consultation mode and added new nonoccupational programs in an attempt to create a system more responsive to individual and corporate needs. Currently, our medical program consists of employment-related physical examinations and direct and preventive health services. The first category includes:

Preemployment physical examinations "by exception" replacing the mandatory physician examination. A registered nurse evaluates the applicant and refers only those applicants who fail a predetermined screening.

Examination to control return to work following illness (three days or more), sick leave, maternity leave, and disability leave. If indicated, a psychological review is also performed.

Complete examination for personnel and their families prior to and after an overseas transfer

Special examination for food handlers to control communicable diseases

Workmen's Compensation examination if injured while at work at a preapproved clinic or by employee's own physician according to Illinois law

Medical care now provided for injury and illness includes:

Diagnosis and initial treatment of trauma to prevent loss of life and/or relieve suffering

Maintenance of records required by various public bodies

First aid training of selected personnel in installations and work shifts that do not have medical personnel in attendance

Counseling to rehabilitate employees troubled by the serious medical-behavioral problems of alcoholism, emotional difficulties, and drug dependencies as well as assistance to overcome other personal crisis caused by marital conflict and legal and financial troubles

Day care facility referral lists for workers with children

Referral list of qualified private physicians

Medical testing in work areas affected by possible outbreak of communicable diseases

Investigation of work areas for possible hazards to a safe and healthful work environment

Consultation with management on medical needs of areas and individual employees if indicated

Active intervention by medical staff toward persons with identified medical problem to encourage treatment and rehabilitation

Individual medical counseling if requested

Obtaining the opinion of a third-party specialist if there is disagreement between our staff and employee's physician on Workmen's Compensation, disability, maternity leave, or sick leave

Preventive health care services now offered include:

Voluntary periodic health examinations for our executive and clerical staffs with eligibility based on age and salary level

Immunization programs for overseas business travel and to prevent outbreaks of influenza. In 1974, 2,500 employees participated; in 1975, 2,275; and in 1976, 1,928 participated

International travel kit containing selected medication to alleviate discomfort of nonserious problems

Health education programs for employees, including education on high blood pressure (921 participated), breast self-examination for cancer (1,878 participated), and eating and heart attack risk (2,045 participated). These programs included a film, models, pamphlets, and a doctor and nurse to answer questions. Two other programs involved brochures and articles in our firm's newspaper: safety and health for summer fun, and venereal disease awareness

These current practices, while an improvement over past practices, have not had the desired impact on our fringe benefit costs; instead, the results were erratic. Medical insurance expenses increased far more than inflation or staff increases would account for; Workmen's Compensation jumped drastically in 1976 as did our paid sick costs; our disability costs decreased until 1976 when they also increased dramatically. The only positive 1976 result was our reduced turnover rate owing to illness/death. (See table 1.) These results indicate that the 1974 reorientation to an occupational medical counseling/consultation mode coupled with new nonoccupational programs needed refinement and further innovation to reduce costs, to meet the ever-changing needs of our employees, and to respond to the increasing legal requirements in the health care area.

Consequently, our future endeavors will encompass a tripartite approach. We intend to upgrade our traditional programs stressing a preventive medical stance coupled with health education. We expect to educate and encourage our personnel to attain a life style that embraces good health practices and prepares them to become knowledgeable health care consumers. To these ends, our future planning encompasses these activities:

Maintain and improve our current medical programs

Redesign and implement a comprehensive safety program to ensure a safe and healthy work environment and control illness and injury on the job

Accelerate management training programs to identify and motivate toward treatment at the earliest stage those employees with personal problems

Provide orientation seminars for employees and families transferring to and from overseas assignments

Offer more health education programs, including smoking clinics, hypertension screening clinics, diabetes detection, weight reduction clinics, and medical articles in the company newspaper delineating good health practices

Outline a nutritional program for the firm's food service areas as well as individual diets for specific medical needs

Offer seminars to reduce and control stress in such areas as vocational needs, marital conflict, divorce, teenage drug abuse, mental health, and child care

Provide a physical fitness facility designed in accordance with aerobics and nutritional concepts to improve the cardiovascular and pulmonary systems

Redesign all data collection systems to ensure more timely data for epidemiological studies to evaluate trends and program effectiveness

Provide health consumer education programs

Table 1.
Fringe Benefit Costs and Selected Outcomes, 1973–1976.

Year	Medical Insurance Cost	Paid Sick Days, Paid Sick Cost	Workmen's Compensation Cost	Disability Cost	Illness + Death Turnover	Average Yearly Staff
1973	$2,148,600	24,329, $747,149	$ 35,957	$360,914	85 + 16 = 101	7,617
1974	2,280,500	23,792, 818,554	52,996	260,373	82 + 21 = 103	7,880
1975	2,669,000	25,568, 931,377	44,753	208,232	67 + 23 = 90	7,948
1976	3,218,752	28,870, 1,128,432	130,443	245,344	59 + 19 = 78	8,071

Planning of Preventive Medical Programs

The employment of preventive medical screening techniques in commercial and industrial settings is quite common nowadays. However, the application of such techniques has been limited in large part to the upper echelons or executive groups. For rank-and-file employees, there are, to be sure, safety regulations, industrial hygiene measurements, and, in certain instances, screening projects for early disease detection. We are aware of several experiments in which corporations have applied preventive medical programs to selected plants or installations. In most instances, these partial efforts have been limited to certain specific goals such as the elimination of stress or early detection of hypertension.

At the Continental Bank, we intend to apply as many as possible of the well-accepted preventive medical principles to our entire work force. This resolve is based partly on altruism, but more importantly on the need to limit costs owing to absenteeism, illness, hospitalization, and downright job maladjustment. We are aware of the magnitude of such a task and approach it with fear and trembling. We recognize that the negative thinkers among our critics could point out obvious shortcomings in such a project. One is the limited impact that can be expected from job-site intervention in a primarily urban, 8,500-person work force. This work force comprises almost 57 percent women and approximately 24 percent blacks, with an age range from the late teens to the middle seventies. Some literature has suggested that women are more resistant to preventive medical efforts than are men. A second problem is the difficulty of inducing permanent changes in behavior patterns. For example, it is a common observation that the overweight worker "goes on the wagon" January 1 or gives up desserts for Lent and drops fifteen or twenty pounds. However, by the time the subsequent winter arrives, he is back up to his original level of obesity. Our hopes are based on the belief that the firm, persistent pressure of education and peer performance may help. However, a third problem is the resentent that such "paternalism" might engender. Again, our educational efforts will be most carefully planned and our suggestions as tactful as possible. We cannot overlook the American tradition of freedom of choice. We imagine that it would be simpler to apply such ideas as we suggest in a German or a Russian factory than in an American bank.

Still another problem is the very great expense of implementing such a program and its educational backup effort. The sad fact is that in most instances, healthy eating is more expensive than "junk food" eating. It is also true that many individuals will exercise only if they are given time off from their job to do so. We recognize these facts but they do not deter us. We feel fortunate that our work force is basically nonunionized; this gives us greater leeway in our planning. Conversely, our program may act to inhibit tendencies toward unionization. We are also aware of the enormous problem of documenting results, measured either in dollars and cents or in a fuller, longer life for our work force. The latter may possibly be reflected in decreased turnover or decreased absenteeism or disability. Inherent in documentation is the establishment and management of a data base. We will touch on these problems in more detail below.

Despite these and other pitfalls, we have decided that the effort should be worthwhile, particularly if we are able to enhance the quality of the employee's life and to forestall the disgruntlement that frequently leads to unionization and high turnover rates. We are also encouraged by the frank commitment of John H. Perkins, president of the bank, who said before a national audience in November 1976:

> To me, the ultimately persuasive argument is the fact that the private sector has three powerful and interrelated economic incentives that make it a humane, but also a discriminating, careful, cost-conscious consumer:
>
> > It must have a stable, reliable, and therefore healthy work force.
> >
> > Consequently, it is willing to pay an affordable premium to help maintain the health of its employees at the same time that it is capable of applying effective administrative and financial management techniques to cost problems of medical care, the health care delivery system, and the needs of employees and the community.
> >
> > As an organic part of the community, the private business finds it imperative—in the interest of its own long-range existence and progress—that the community itself have available a cost-effective health care structure of the highest quality.
>
> Every human life carries with it an obligation to maintain its health to the best of its ability, and I believe that the awareness of this obligation is the essence of health care consumerism. It is this personal awareness that must be broadened and elevated to the level of an integrated community endeavor. Once this condition is achieved—and there are community examples to indicate that it can be—it is possible to bring costs under control without damaging either the existing health care system or the recipients of the care.

Thus, we fools will tiptoe where angels have mostly feared to tread into the areas of personal life style. In the area of nutrition, most emphatically, we make no claims for originality. The occupational medical scene today is studded with examples of excellent nutritional projects and studies. In addition, government sponsored programs, such as the MR FIT and Coronary Prevention studies, certainly have provided a solid groundwork for our venture. On the other hand, we doubt that the techniques that can be established for one workplace, such as our bank, can be applied to larger masses of people in a study like Coronary Prevention, a community like Framingham, or a territory like Karelia. We will offer separate menus to our employees with specific recommendations for calorie limitation, avoidance of excess animal fats, foods regarded as beneficial to the intestinal tract, and other considerations. We will experiment with motivational methods, including price advantages, experimental food preparation techniques, and lotteries. In addition, a single module of our work force will be eating in a newly constructed atrium-like, plant-surrounded cafeteria that is quite unlike most of those we are familiar with in the industrial plants and commercial concerns of this country. In this setting, we hope to eliminate stress from the eating place. A factor that may or may not be in our favor is that many of our workers, both those in the lower income groups and those at the management level, tend to make the noon meal at Continental Bank their main source of nutrition and calories. We think that this fact will make more efficacious our interventions and give us more leverage than would be possible in population groups where the main meal is at home in the evening with the family.

In our exercise and physical fitness program, we will emphasize the hygenic aspects of physical activity like walking, calisthenics, and other activities. The question of implementing more strenuous competitive exercise such as racquetball, handball, and so on, is continually before our minds but not as yet resolved. We visualize eventually making exercise facilities of one kind or another available to anyone who works for the bank. At present, however, it does not seem feasible to offer these facilities while the worker is expected to be on the job, but motivational techniques may also be applicable to this problem. With regard to the single module of our work force mentioned above, an exercise area is already beyond the blueprint stage. This facility will have lockers, showers, a treadmill for exercise prescriptions, trained attendants, and, of course, capability for accommodating both men and women.

Although the physical aspects of stress in a bank atmosphere seem of less concern than in heavy industry, we recognize that a number of jobs have important stress factors attached; in others, boredom is a serious obstacle to performance. In addition, the dissatisfied employee or mismatched manager is a point of stress in any work situation. Our educational efforts with management will make evident our concern in this area. Consultants have been and will continue to be utilized to analyze emotional and psychological stress factors in our workplace, and active efforts will be made to control them. We are particularly concerned with the high incidence of emotional difficulties and adjustment problems in the young black mothers of our work force. Many of these women carry the burden of their family's care, nutrition, and housing along with the obligation to earn a living. Relief of such situations, or amelioration thereof, will be a specific target of our counseling section. In addition, it is our thesis that particularly long or difficult commutes can be exceedingly stressful. Finally, the ever-increasing size of our overseas work force imposes stresses on entire families of those employees who must pull up their roots to live in a foreign land. We will intervene in such instances when they are identified and seem amenable to manipulation.

We will also be concerned with the correction of factors thought to cause degenerative cardiovascular disease and other major killers. In an attempt to control hypertension, the Medical Department will monitor (and advise treatment where necessary) the blood pressure of all employees shown to elevated blood pressure by routine screening procedures. The blood fats, including cholesterol and triglycerides, are now monitored in our managerial population and in a significant portion of our nonmanagerial work force. It is our intention to expand these screening programs and to work educationally in programs such as those described above to convince all employees of the importance of prophylactic measures in the prevention of premature cardiovascular disease. Other medical measures, including correction of obesity, diabetes detection, common preventive medical techniques, and psychological services, will be applied as indicated.

Cigarette smoking will be the object of intense, firm, unremitting pressure from our group. It has not been possible so far to achieve a ban on smoking among employees while on the job in the bank. It does not seem realistic to hope to accomplish this entirely in the future. On the other hand, the overwhelming data indicating that cigarettes are a direct killer will be continuously presented to the work force through more energetic techniques than most employers would utilize.

The vital problem of data collection has been a central element of our planning. To this point, the following pertinent items have been included in our human resources data base:

Basic Data

    Name
    Date of birth
    Address (zip code)
    Sex
    Race
    Handicap code
    Selective Service status

Employment Data

    Data entered service
    Interviewer code
    Source of referral

Job Data

    Current job title
    Date on current job

Education Data

    Years of education code
    Highest degree, date, school, major
    Degree currently sought, expected date, school, major

Salary Administration Data

    Current salary or hourly rate
    6 previous salary increases: amount, date, type
    Performance rating
    Potential rating

Benefits Data

    Blood program cycle code
    Health insurance option
    Dental coverage

We also propose to add certain elements that may or may not prove difficult to obtain. These include head of household, ownership of automobile, smoking habit, and perhaps even general physical fitness category. These data may eventually give us a basis for suspecting the health effects of certain life styles that are not amenable to direct measurement.

With regard to data, there is still another serious problem. This is the question of availability of medical care as it varies in the two options for health care delivery (HMO versus fee-for-service). To interpret the effects of these in our system, it will be necessary to achieve wholehearted cooperation from the insurance carriers. To this point, it has not been the habit of Blue Cross or Blue Shield to supply detailed morbidity and mortality data. However, we are hopeful that we will be able to persuade them to provide the necessary information. We feel that a period of at least five years will be necessary for collection and correlation of data before we can make any statements about the positive or negative effects of our attempted interventions.

Particular attention will be devoted to educating our employees for their role as health care consumers.

The Health Care Consumer Education Program

To be a wise consumer of health care services, a person should purchase only necessary or desirable services at a price that is reasonable and fair, and should have some control over the services while they are rendered coupled with appropriate channels for later recourse to personally assured high quality care. To accomplish this the consumer needs to gather considerable information starting when a course of treatment is being planned. Thus, health consumer education has two main elements. The first is to sensitize employees to their role as patients in treatment decisions. Their personal responsibility must be emphasized recurrently with articles in the house newspaper, leaflets for general distribution, and the employee handbook. The second element is specific information on need, desirability, price, and expectable outcome of alternative plans for treatment of a diagnosed condition.

The role of patient entails the personal responsibility to authorize or accept any and all forms of treatment. It is the patient's decision whether to take medication. It is the patient's authorization that allows surgery. Without the patient's approval, the practice of medicine is against the law. If the patient truly realizes and accepts this responsibility for medical treatment decisions and is given enough time, he or she will make better decisions based on multiple sources of information and his or her own personal values. This involves treating the medical professional as an adviser rather than an authority. The wise consumer will consider doctor's advice rather than follow doctor's orders.

In this context, surgical services deserve special attention. Unlike other forms of treatment involving medication, diet, rest, or exercise, surgery once administered cannot be modified or reversed if it proves to be wrong or unnecessary. Therefore, the patient must be sure that surgery is the single best solution to a problem before it is authorized. A program of referral and insurance coverage for additional surgical opinions can help the patient gather information about the necessity of surgery. On May 1, 1977, the health insurance claim representatives in our personnel office began to consult with employees and their family members on surgery decisions. Those who would like more information before they agree to surgery are given a list of three certified specialists who have enrolled in Chicago Blue Cross–Blue Shield's experimental second opinion program. The second doctor may be consulted with or without the first doctor's knowledge. The patient is free to seek a third opinion if the second disagrees with the recommended surgery. There is no cost to the patient for the additional opinions, and the expense of the surgery will be covered even if it is not recommended by the second and third opinions. The expectation is that the additional cost of diagnosis will be more than repaid in savings from avoided surgery and hospitalization.

It is fairly clear that patients will be concerned about the price of their personal medical services only if they share some of the cost. This fact, coupled with the perception that price and care quality are directly related, may lead the patient to feel more assured and satisfied with higher costs. However, when insurance plans cover doctors' fees only as a percentage of "usual and custom-ary" or "reasonable and customary" charges, the patient can have an unwel-come surprise after the insurance company pays the claim. For example, if a doctor charges $800 for a procedure and usual and customary for this proce-dure is $400, the insurance plan covering 80 percent of usual and customary charges would pay $320. The patient finds that his or her share of the $800 bill is $480 rather than $160, or 20 percent of the $800.

By this time the doctor is beyond reproach. He or she has saved the life of the patient who is now inclined to attack the "skimpy" insurance plan and the employer. The patient has found out the doctor's fee and how much of it his insurance will cover too late to do anything. By agreeing to have the treatment, the patient has tacitly agreed to pay the doctor's fee with or without the insurance coverage. Usual and customary fees can function as an effective restraint on physicians' charges only if the patient is able to compare the doctor's fee with usual and customary beforehand.

On June 1, 1977, our health insurance claim representatives began to determine the impact of usual and customary charges in advance. To make use of this service, employees must first obtain detailed price and treatment plan information from the physician. Many people consider this bad form, but our health education program will point out that they may be surprised after the fact by what the insurance pays. Thus motivated by an uncertain personal expenditure, a person will be encouraged to ask the doctor beforehand. The employee can come to our employee benefit office with a written statement of the fee and procedure and find out how much, if any, of that fee will be beyond usual and customary limits. This, then, will provide him or her with informa-tion by which to judge the doctor's price.

When employees come to our health insurance claim representatives for second surgical opinions or predetermination of usual and customary charge limit impact, they can also be counseled on ways to control the quality of care. First, they must learn all they can about the nature of their illness, various treatment modes, and ways to prevent a recurrence. Just as patients must approve a plan of treatment, they also may accept or refuse any part of a treatment program. Therefore, patients can review health services while care is in progress. First, they can select the day of admission to the hospital and try to avoid going Friday or Saturday for surgical procedures to be conducted on Monday or Tuesday. They can seek to understand why they need each medica-tion or supply and what it will do by consulting with their doctor and nurses. Generic drugs can be requested. The patient may want to watch the "checkout time" when it comes time for discharge, to avoid charges for another day in the hospital.

Later on, we plan to implement a utilization review program with the

Chicago Foundation for Medical Care. Assuming a well person does not want to stay in a hospital, employees may be able to use statistics on expected length of stay to monitor their own progress and plan for discharge. This will be possible through disclosure of the current length-of-stay review to the patient. Admittedly, this program will have more meaning if hospital costs are shared between the insurer and the patient. For it to be clearly in the patient's interest to be cost conscious about the use of hospital care, the hospital must cost him or her more than substitutable outpatient services.

A New Corporate Prepaid Group Health Plan

Bynum E. Tudor

An omnibus, prepaid health care program for employees has been established by R. J. Reynolds Industries, Inc., in its headquarters city of Winston-Salem, North Carolina. This program represents the most extensive private health care commitment on the part of a corporate employer since the organization of the Kaiser-Permanente system in California more than thirty years ago. It is an outpatient, closed-panel health maintenance organization (HMO) designed to accomodate the full spectrum of employee health needs, using all preventive, diagnostic, pharmaceutical, surgical, and therapeutic means available. Started on July 1, 1976, with a membership of 6,000, it has grown to a current enrollment of 10,000, and projections are that the maximum level of 30,000 members will be attained within three years. It is estimated that 85 percent of R. J. Reynolds' 15,000 Winston-Salem employees ultimately will belong to the plan.

The plan is headquartered in a new, 37,000-square-foot health care center equipped with a complete range of basic diagnostic, laboratory, and records facilities. A staff of sixty-eight is presently on hand to serve the members, comprising five internists, four pediatricians, one obstetrician-gynecologist, six physicians' assistants or nurse practitioners, twenty allied health technicians, and an administrative support complement of thirty-two. It is expected that the plan will have doubled its number of physicians to twenty by the end of 1977. Full provision is made for referring patients to any needed specialists, and staff physicians have admissions privileges at Winston-Salem's three major hospitals. Emergency and ambulance service is also furnished through agreement with these hospitals.

Treatment is not limited to local resources, however. R. J. Reynolds is willing to draw upon whatever nationwide or worldwide capabilities are needed, to the extent of flying patients to treatment by the most eminent medical authorities, or bringing these authorities themselves to Winston-Salem. Evidence of this willingness was displayed last year when a Hong Kong employee of an R. J. Reynolds subsidiary was flown to Stanford University in Palo Alto, California, for open-heart surgery, and was accompanied by two attending specialists and two registered nurses.

All bills are paid by R. J. Reynolds and there are no claim forms for employees to fill out. The only charge to employees is a token three-dollar monthly fee for dependents and a one-dollar handling fee per prescription, under a system honored by nearly all Winston-Salem drug stores. Coverage of employees away from home has been arranged by R. J. Reynolds through Equitable Insurance Company. Expenses associated with any catastrophes that might occur will be handled by R. J. Reynolds directly from the company treasury: the firm registered $5.75 billion in sales and revenues in 1976 and lists current assests of more than $2 billion. Although only R. J. Reynolds employees are eligible for the new health care program, known formally as Winston-Salem Health Care Plan, Inc., the HMO has been chartered by the state of North Carolina as a nonprofit organization, legally independent of the company.

Still, R. J. Reynolds considers the HMO a functional extension of its $195 million employee benefits program. R. J. Reynolds' vice-president serves as president and chairman of the board of directors of Winston-Salem Health Care Plan, the corporate director of employee benefits has been instrumental in the creation of Winston-Salem Health Care Plan and functions as vice-president and treasurer; the company's manager of employee benefits serves as secretary of the HMO.

Although R. J. Reynolds is the only corporation involved with Winston-Salem Health Care Plan, other area firms did have an opportunity to participate from the beginning. Some of them were represented on a ten-member Winston-Salem Chamber of Commerce ad hoc committee, chaired by Reynolds' corporate director of employee benefits, that was formed more than six years ago to investigate region-wide solutions to health care problems. However, when after several years of study the committee decided that formation of a controlled HMO was the most appropriate direction to take, R. J. Reynolds was the only area company that stood as an effective advocate of the idea.

As a result, R. J. Reynolds has financed the plan by itself. The company in 1974 paid out $1.2 million for the unfinished shell of a two-story office building in an industrial park just off a freeway on the west side of Winston-Salem. The deal included a three-and-a-half-acre tract of land that could serve for future expansion. R. J. Reynolds backed up this expenditure by allocating another $1 million for new diagnostic, laboratory, and records facilities, as well as for a complete interior design. The company is in the process of adding a $200,000 outside elevator to the health care center, to cap off the major capital outlays.

If R. J. Reynolds was the only Winston-Salem company to favor the HMO, perhaps the company had more compelling reasons than neighboring firms. A direct impetus came in 1972, when R. J. Reynolds was in the process of relocating the headquarters of RJR Foods, the company's convenience foods and beverages subsidiary, from New York to Winston-Salem. The move involved more than 100 persons, and in helping RJR Foods' families resettle in the community, one of the company's tasks was to find medical services for them.

It was then that R. J. Reynolds discovered surprising shortage of access to quality health care within the community. Although Winston-Salem is the home of the Bowman Gray School of Medicine of Wake Forest University, one of the best-known medical education institutions in the nation, and although the city has a high number of physicians per capita, it was found that many area doctors were engaged in teaching or research and were not in family practice.

Further investigation by R. J. Reynolds revealed that about 50 percent of the company's existing Winston-Salem employees did not have a family physician. Instead, they were using the emergency rooms of local hospitals for all visits, emergency and nonemergency. R. J. Reynolds found that one local hospital emergency room during a single year had treated 70,000 nonemergency complaints. Of course, there was no way to determine how many of these were company employees or their dependents, but it was apparent that a large number were.

The company realized that this situation carried manifold implications. Obviously, the city's emergency rooms were being misused, and were constantly being tied up by people with noncritical injuries and ailments. The company reasoned that this circumstance had to impair the ability of the emergency rooms to handle the truly urgent cases. Another aspect of the problem was that employee use of emergency room doctors as surrogate family physicians represented heightened medical costs. Standard emergency room fees were about double the going rate charged by area physicians in private practice.

R. J. Reynolds decided to make a thorough scrutiny of its employee-related medical expenses and came up with some salient findings. Company records showed that far from being cost minimizers, Blue Cross–Blue Shield carried a built-in bias toward increased hospitalization of employees. R. J. Reynolds' corporate health insurance package provided that employees receive greater insurance compensation for hospitalization than for visits to doctors' offices or to outpatient facilities. As a result, the company uncovered such glaring excesses as a woman employee being hospitalized for forty-five days for routine treatment that should have lasted ten days. With local hospital charges running about $200 a day, the extra cost was around $7,000. Owing in part to this kind of immoderation, company medical premium expenses had been rising 20 percent each year since 1970.

Compounding the difficulty was the fact that both hospital expenses and physicians' fees were outpacing normal inflation. Because Blue Cross–Blue Shield neither had any incentive to reduce these expenses nor cared to touch the traditionally hallowed doctor-patient relationship, the main cost control element was missing. A little more investigation by the company uncovered various other sources of pressure toward inflation of medical costs. For one thing, recent years have brought forth an impressive array of advances in various surgical and rehabilitative techniques and facilities, and physicians and hospitals are continually being encouraged to implement them. Hospitals often are nonprofit institutions directed by lay boards, determined that their medical facility will contain nothing but the best, regardless of cost. Their experience has been that the government and the insurance providers, who control 92 percent of medical spending in the United States, have always been willing to foot the bill, with few questions asked.

Most hospitals, too, have excess bed capacity, and find it mandatory to keep that filled in order to remain solvent and defray their heavy overhead costs. So, they cater to physicians, who control the who and what of hospital admissions. Hospitals court the doctors with the latest in costly surgical and laboratory equipment and large staffs of professional and support personnel. (It is estimated that labor constitutes 70 percent of hospital costs.)

Doctors have not been blameless, either. The amount of unnecessary surgery performed annually in this nation has been termed "a national disgrace" by the Federal Register, which cites expert opinion that 20–50 percent of all operations are unneeded. In addition, soaring malpractice premiums have instilled a great fear in doctors, many of whom have tended to protect themselves by ordering extra tests to substantiate their diagnosis. Several leading medical authorities decry these extra tests as needless, overly expensive, and of little value to patients. One of the dissenters has observed that a doctor, being 95 percent sure of a diagnosis, might order another dozen expensive tests so that he might be 98 percent sure.

This cost spiral gave R. J. Reynolds a final push toward creation of an HMO, with its emphasis on financial control and preventive medicine. The company decided that the traditional priorities of medicine had been misplaced, that doctors should be rewarded more for keeping people well, rather than so much for treating them when they are sick.

Results of this first nine months of operation of Winston-Salem Health Care Plan indicate that the HMO is working well in the primary areas of preventive medicine and reduction of hospitalization. Whereas R. J. Reynolds had experienced more than 900 days of hospitalization per 1,000 employees annually just before the HMO was established, members of Winston-Salem Health Care Plan have been hospitalized at a rate of 436 per 1,000. This record is an impressive one in light of the fact that many new members had avoided paying for a $125 physical examination, and waited for a physical at the Winston-Salem Health Care Plan to turn up any maladies. The HMO staff reports, in fact, that many members had not undergone a physical examination for years.

Realizing that some employees, especially the older ones, would want to retain their long-standing family physician, R. J. Reynolds continues to offer its standard Blue Cross–Blue Shield package as an alternative to HMO membership. But by using claims monitoring and other review means, R. J. Reynolds has been able to reduce to 681 per 1,000 the hospitalization rate of those still covered by Blue Cross–Blue Shield.

If it were to continue its present performance, R. J. Reynolds' HMO might move out of debt within eighteen months—half the originally forecast break-even period of three to four years. Of course, exactly what constitutes "breaking even" is difficult to judge, owing to the various capital and start-up costs absorbed in the first months of operation. The operators of the HMO feel it will take twenty-four months to develop realistic figures.

Some of these one-time, beginning expenses involved recruiting, because the caliber of the medical staff is the pivotal aspect of any new health care program. R. J. Reynolds' HMO achieved a running start when Dr. E. Reid Bahnson, a Wake Forest professor and past president of the home Forsyth County Medical Society, agreed to become medical director of the plan. Dr. Bahnson not only managed to forestall any local misgivings about the formation of the HMO, but was able to draw upon valuable contacts at leading medical schools and hospitals throughout the nation.

Consequently, there has been no dearth of applications by professionals wanting affiliation with Winston-Salem Health Care Plan. The search for a full-time professional administrator ended when Donald Hurst, who had headed an HMO for a major oil company for a number of years, agreed to take the position in January 1975. Mr. Hurst quickly became involved in comprehensive long-range planning for the HMO. Altogether, Dr. Bahnson, Mr. Hurst, and other HMO administrators have evaluated more than 1,000 applications and have interviewed over 170 professionals to fill the 20 physicians' spots within the current staff quota. Given this wide selection, Dr. Bahnson and his colleagues have been able to apply some exacting criteria. One automatic requirement is that a physician be either board-certified or board-qualified. Educational backgrounds and subspecialities have been carefully examined. After Dr. Bahnson is satisfied with a candidate, that doctor is invited to meet the chiefs of staff within his specialty at each of Winston-Salem's three major hospitals. If all chiefs of staff agree that the doctor can have admitting privileges, then Winston-Salem Health Care Plan will ordinarily make the physician an offer. Since the managers of the HMO have resolved that physicians' salaries are certainly an area in which they will not scrimp, the offer is usually a very competitive one. It is the feeling at Winston-Salem Health Care Plan that the member physicians should receive remuneration that is in the top half of what their peers receive.

The experience has been that many doctors are willing to join an HMO for reasons other than the monetary. Many want to escape the distractions and annoyances of having to manage a business—mundane chores that occupy up to 35 percent of the time of a private practitioner. Working at an HMO also enables a physician to work a set schedule, obtain corporate fringe benefits and paid vacation and holidays, enjoy the "cover" of his colleagues during off-hours, and avoid malpractice insurance worries. With these various inducements attracting high-caliber professionals, the Winston-Salem Health Care Plan has been able to strike a desirable balance in the mix of its staff—a number of older, more experienced doctors offset by younger doctors with the newer techniques fresh in mind.

The situation has also made it possible for Winston-Salem Health Care Plan to plan its staffing levels carefully according to anticipated membership growth and specialty needs. Close track is being kept of all referrals—their results and their costs. By using these data and by consulting with Dr. Bahnson, R. J. Reynolds can evaluate charges by procedure and will be able to effectively control long-run costs. The statistics will be made into annualized figures that and compared with accepted HMO guidelines, signaling when to hire a specialist rather than continue costly referrals. For instance, the common rule of thumb is that there should be an internist for every 3,000 members in such a group plan and a pediatrician for every 5,000 members. A plan might need 10,000 members to justify the addition of an ophthamologist, who is a particularly high-paid specialist. Monitoring of patient load during the first nine months of activity at Winston-Salem Health Care Plan has shown some patterns that do not fit these national norms, but it might take twenty-four months to determine whether the patterns will right themselves, or to isolate some local idiosyncrasies. Generally, though, the developers of Winston-Salem Health Care Plan believe that a membership of 30,000 is the minimum that can support a representative medical staff with true economies of scale.

Actually, Winston-Salem Health Care Plan has chosen to overstaff slightly for the first months of operation. New members have heard much persuasion and promotion regarding an HMO and its services, and nothing deflates their expectations more than having to wait hours past their appointment or receive a cursory examination because the medical team is understaffed and overworked. There is no faster way to lose competent physicians and waste expensive recruiting efforts, either. Thanks to overstaffing at Winston-Salem Health Care Plan, initial patients have encountered a minimum of waiting (fifteen minutes is the target limit) and staff physicians have been able to give the utmost in personal attention to them.

This tactic is part of an overall philosophy that the R. J. Reynolds HMO, being the first of its kind in the Southeast, represents such a drastically different form of health care delivery that members will have to be continually educated on the benefits of the arrangement. Then, goes the theory, they in turn will tell their friends and fellow employees and the popularity of the program will spread throughout R. J. Reynolds.

Even the decor of the new health care center is considered part of the educational process. A professional interior decorator, who had never dealt with medical environments before, was brought in to produce a look that was different from the sterile sterotypes. He created a contemporary design that makes liberal use of textured wallpaper and curtains, framed artwork, and cushioned bamboo furniture. The motif is carried throughout the center, from reception areas to nurses' and appointments stations to doctors' offices and examining rooms, to instill an atmosphere of maximum physical and mental relaxation for the members. The educational technique has worked well enough that one patient recently arrived at a reception room complaining of a headache and fifteen minutes later said he wanted to go home because he felt better.

It is this human side to setting up its own HMO that has appealed to R. J. Reynolds the most. When the medical staff at Winston-Salem Health Care Plan detects something like high blood sugar or hypertension in a patient and is able to treat the condition before it turns worse, the value in human terms is inestimable. The company fully realizes that when any member of an employee's household is sick, it can affect that employee's entire outlook, both on and off the job. On the other hand, the personalized brand of preventive medicine stressed by the HMO serves to insulate employees and their families from needless infirmities and distress, and undoubtedly prolongs their lives.

Word-of-mouth about the pleasant environs and personalized treatment at Winston-Salem Health Care Plan has evidently moved throughout the company, because more employees are asking to join the HMO every week. There was such a deluge of requests during the first membership drive that the company resorted to computerized selection as an impartial method of enrollment. Members were selected randomly, but only after the computer was programmed to develop a membership that was representative of the total R. J. Reynolds employee population, in terms of age, sex, race, position, seniority, and so on. This not only makes for a completely equitable arrangement and heads off possible hard feelings, but enables the company to properly analyze treatment at the HMO. It is known, for instance, there will not be an unusual number of tonsilectomies because there are not many five- and six-year-olds enrolled, or disproportionate numbers with arthritis because there is not an extreme number of older folks in the program.

The utilization of the HMO was unexpectedly heavy from the first day. Inasmuch as the opening was in July, the belief prevailed that many members would be on vacation or would postpone visits in favor of outdoor activities. It was also thought there would be an initial restraint in trying out the new concept. Instead, members turned out to be curious enough to want to test the HMO's services immediately. It also seems that many had delayed taking physical examinations and inquiring about assorted aches and pains once they learned they had been accepted into the plan. Fortunately, the above-mentioned overstaffing was able to pull the Winston-Salem Health Care Plan through its initial trials.

There were surprisingly few complaints from the start, especially considering that people often are used to one doctor and find it hard to adjust to the ways of a new one. It was also anticipated that some members would be confused by their first experience with being administered to by a nurse practitioner or physicians assistant, but patients have received these two new types of medical personnel uneventfully.

One reason that the R. J. Reynolds HMO has done well initially is that the plan is modeled after the best features of the most successful HMOs in the nation. A team of six company investigators spent hundreds of overtime and weekend hours visiting successful HMOs throughout the nation. They even made return trips to view programs in such scattered locations as New York, Arizona, Connecticut, Oregon, and Ohio. Studies of the HMOs at Harvard University, New Haven, Connecticut, and Rochester, New York, as well as the Kaiser system, were especially fruitful. R. J. Reynolds also used the services of the Group Health Association of America in Washington, D.C., to gain vital facts, figures, and contacts, and consulted the Department of Health, Education, and Welfare office in Rockville, Maryland, to glean the results of broader studies.

Two of the more valuable lessons learned through this process were that an HMO should restrict initial enrollment, and, in the corporate situation, should ask the chief executive officer of the firm to give public sanction to the program. R. J. Reynolds Industries Chairman Colin Stokes readily assented to the second point. When Mr. Stokes' endorsement of the Winston-Salem Health Care Plan was carried widely by area media, the program received a direct boost.

The initial ceiling on membership also created interest in the HMO, in a sort of inverse manner. R. J. Reynolds' earlier investigations had shown that some HMOs had thrown their membership wide open and suffered for it. People seem to hold cheaply anything that comes too easily, regardless of its intrinsic value. The HMOs that had been nonrestrictive realized only a fraction of their needed enrollment, their facilities sat idle, overhead became unbearable, and the ventures failed. Other HMOs that limited initial enrollment gained a tantalizing aura of exclusivity and heard from as many prospective members as they wanted.

These same HMOs also served as models of how to best manage a health care delivery system containing thousands of members. Winston-Salem Health Care Plan has borrowed some of their methods to build a comprehensive computerized records bank at its health care center, maintaining a complete medical history on every member. The computer system is linked to the telephone system within the HMO facility, so that any staff physician may make an entry into the files merely by calling it in. Files are accessible to the physicians within a moment's notice, of course, and are delivered to them automatically before a patient's appointment. Files are updated following all appointments and after any patient test results become known.

Significantly, the computer is also employed to generate weekly reports covering a broad cross section of treatment work, including patient load by doctor, and so on. These reports are used by the medical director to monitor the performances of the doctors and the laboratories at the same time, to make sure that a particular doctor is not loading up the laboratories with unnecessary testing, and to confirm that the laboratories are producing their findings swiftly and accurately. The use of surgery by physicians in the Winston-Salem Health Care Plan also is tightly monitored. Staff doctors are directed to make sparing use of surgery. Before any surgery is contemplated, the full medical team confers about it, making a complete review of the patient's medical history and recent testing and exploring all alternatives to surgery. If they finally do agree that an operation is necessary, only then is the patient informed.

R. J. Reynolds believes that HMOs, by demonstrating this type of heightened respect for patient self-interest, will become increasingly well-known and that the majority of thinking people will want to join them. HMOs are, after all, the leading alternative in the offing to the national health care system, and indeed may be the only hope of rescue from what may well be another massive fiasco on the part of the government. Surely the same people who made such a botch of Medicare and Medicaid cannot be expected but to fail on even a larger scale with national health insurance.

Since those in the private sector are going to be spending large amounts of money for health care one way or another, it becomes incumbent on corporations to investigate the HMO alternative seriously, if for no other reason than to be in control of the expenditures. When it comes to spending the stockholders' money on employee relations, the HMO makes much more sense than such nonproductive categories as pensions, increased holidays or vacations, or other added fringe benefits. HMOs give business a chance to insure a happy and effective work force, reduce absenteeism and downtime, promote efficiency, and reduce annual expenditures for sick pay.

R. J. Reynolds considers HMOs the trend of the future in national health care delivery. The company has received some 120 corporate inquiries about its HMO, including many from other Fortune 500 companies, and knows of 7 major firms that plan to closely emulate the Winston-Salem Health Care Plan arrangement. R. J. Reynolds stands ready to aid such plans in every way possible, in hopes of matching the cooperation the company received during the development of is own HMO.

TRENDS

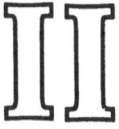

A Classification of Seven Corporate Health Clinics

Mark C. Schofield and Richard H. Egdahl

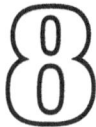

Seven industrial clinics in the greater Boston area have been surveyed and a classification scheme developed by level and type of services provided. The kind of clinic established appears to depend both upon a firms's resources and on the way in which management perceives a clinic's role in relation to the health care delivery system as a whole. Now is an advantageous time to undertake such a study since increased responsibilities under the Occupational Safety and Health Act have stimulated expansion of clinics in some industries, and informed speculation suggests that this trend will continue.[1] The imperative to expand services comes at a time when the rising cost of health care has caused industry to reexamine its investment in employee health. Although decreasing unnecessary hospitalization has been a major theme in industry's cost control efforts,[2] less attention has been paid to the role of industry's own health clinic in striving for cost containment and health enhancement.

The survey is intended as a first step in an analysis of the role that industrial clinics currently play in health care delivery. It is possible that programs can be developed and expanded in these clinics that will provide the basis for effecting improvements in health services both for employees and for their families.

In order to assess current patterns of care delivered by industrial clinics, advantages perceived by firms that provide health services for employees, and attitudes toward expansion of industrial clinic services, interviews were conducted with health care providers from seven firms in the greater Boston area. The sample includes representatives of several types of industries: manufacturing, finance, communications, and energy. The firms also vary in the number of workers they employ (600–35,000), although the majority fall within the 4,000–6,000 range. Two of the firms are unionized. Two companies were selected because they were known to have active and innovative employee health care programs.

Most information was obtained in personal interviews; follow-up telephone interviews were used for supplementary information. An effort was made to include in the personal interview the manager responsible for clinic policy and employee health benefits and the physician in charge of the clinic. In some cases, this was not possible to arrange, as, for example, where the medical department is a separate organizational entity. The medical director in these cases serves a dual role as a clinic manager and a provider of health services. An effort was made to talk with as many persons as necessary to obtain a clear picture of clinic policy and function.

The interviews lasted from one to two hours and covered a wide variety of health-related topics. They opened with a series of questions on basic services, staffing patterns, clinic policies, and special programs. An effort was then made to delineate the broad outlines of clinic policy and their financial and service justifications. Finally, reaction to possible future expansion of clinic services was sought.

Although anonymity was not a precondition of the interviews, the firms are not identified. The information is presented in tables and case studies. The case study format was used because it most closely reflects the way in which the information was gathered. Despite the variety of the sample, selection procedures were not rigorously controlled and caution should be used in generalizing from the results. All firms face the dilemma of rising health care costs, but each firm's response springs from its particular circumstances. Therefore, much practical knowledge can be gained from evaluating the bases for development of policies and programs of individual firms. However, the policies and health programs of the firms represented in this sample are not necessarily typical of industry as a whole.

The findings from the survey portion of the interviews are recorded in tables 1, 2 and 3. Table 1 includes a general description of the firms in the sample and their clinic facilities and services. The column labeled "policy of employee care" contains a brief statement of the types of care offered. The firms are listed roughly according to the extent of their involvement in nonoccupational health care (with firms A, B and C offering primarily occupational care and F and G offering complete primary care services). It should be assumed, therefore, that types of care provided by clinics at the top of the table are also provided by the clinics in the latter portion of the table (for example, Firms F

Table 1.
Firm and Clinic Characteristics.

Firm	Number Employed	Policy of Employee Care	Nonroutine Services	Facilities	Classification
A—light manufacturing	600	care for occupational injuries and illnesses; routine primary care services discouraged	physicals: yearly for management, yearly for employees over 40, biannually for employees under 40; monthly health seminars	dispensary-type, EKG	occupational
B—manufacturing	4,000	same as A with emphasis on emergency care	flu innoculation, executive physicals (through an outside agency)	clinic-type	occupational
C—finance	5,400	same as A	yearly executive physicals, flu innoculations, shots for foreign travel, allergy, desensitization shots, hearing and vision testing	clinic-type, EKG	occupational

[Continued]

Table 1. [Continued]
Firm and Clinic Characteristics.

Firm	Number Employed	Policy of Employee Care	Nonrountine Services	Facilities	Classification
D—manufacturing	4,000	primary emphasis on treatment and prevention of industrial accidents; open-door sick call, some diagnostic and primary care services offered	yearly management physicals, voluntary employee physicals, flu innoculation, lab work and x-ray at cost for nonoccupational testing, hearing testing	clinic-type, laboratory, x-ray	mixed
E—communications	35,000[a]	care for occupational injuries and illnesses; some diagnostic, preventive, and primary care services	physicals for employees over 35, x-ray and lab when ordered by a company physician or requested by private physician, short-term nonoccupational care, retirement counseling, hearing, vision, and pulmonary function testing	clinic-type, laboratory, x-ray, computerized medical record system, EKG	mixed

F—utility	4,000	care for occupational injuries; open-door sick call	physicals: annually to employees over 50, biannually to employees 30–50, triannually for employees under 30; primary care and diagnostic services, hearing and vision testing, pulmonary function testing	clinic-type, laboratory, EKG, x-ray (by contract with outside service)	comprehensive
G—manufacturing	6,000	total health care[b]	annual physicals; primary care and diagnostic services for all employees; eyeglasses; vision, hearing, and pulmonary function testing	clinic-type, laboratory, EKG	comprehensive

[a]30,000 within range of clinic.
[b]Self-description.

and G do provide occupational care although it is not listed). The next column, entitled "nonroutine services provided," lists non occupational services provided by the firms (routine services offered by all the clinics such as preemployment physical examination and screening programs are excluded). Such items as hearing and vision testing are included in this column although they may be offered exclusively as part of the preemployment exam. The next column labeled "facilities" contains two items of information. First the health care facility is classified either as a "clinic-type" or a "dispensary-type." The facilities described here as of the clinic-type contain several examining rooms, an employee waiting area and occasionally an employee holding area, or laboratory and x-ray facilities. The dispensary-type facilities are generally more limited, having fewer examining rooms and less ancillary space. Finally, under the general heading "facilities" are included laboratory, x-ray, and EKG testing.

The final item included in table 2 (labeled "classification") requires a more detailed explanation. The clinics are classified into three groups based on the broad outlines of policy governing services made available to employees. Occupational clinics deliver care for emergencies, occupational injuries, and illnesses that occur when the employee is at work. Comprehensive clinics deliver a much wider range of health services. The two clinics included in this category have "open-door" policies: employees are allowed to visit the clinic for any complaint, and the clinic is the sole source of care for some of them. The mixed-clinic category includes those having policies broadly resembling those of the occupational clinics, but which offer some nonoccupational services. The case studies of the clinics are arranged according to this classification scheme.

The following "case studies" are condensations of more detailed descriptions of the health care programs written after the interviews. An effort was made to supplement the information provided in the tables as well as capture the special features of each firm's program.

Firm A has the smallest number of employees among the firms studied. Furthermore, the number of employees has been decreasing in recent years, limiting the firm's ability to experiment with innovative health care programs. At the time of the interview Firm A's parent corporation was in the process of reevaluating its employee health benefits policy. Several innovative insurance programs have been considered, but a representative stated that the most practical option would probably be to recommend increasing employee contributions to health insurance premiums. This was recognized as a temporary solution, but it appeared to be the only practical alternative given the firm's size and satisfaction with its current benefit package.

Employee health care is provided at a dispensary-type clinic staffed by three part-time physicians and a full-time nurse. During the past year a new nurse was hired and the traditional role of plant nurse was expanded to include employee health education and occupational safety and health duties, including OSHA responsibilities. An electronic paging system allows the nurse freedom of movement in the plant while permitting her to be reached in emergencies.

The firm hires two part-time physicians for a total of twenty-three hours per month. Time limitations demand that the physicians' activities be restricted primarily to physical examinations; nonoccupational care is discouraged.

In addition to the two primary care physicians, the firm also contracts for the services of a part-time (one half-day per week) psychiatrist, who conducts training programs for supervisors and management personnel and provides referral services for employees seeking psychiatric consultation. This latter service provides management with an overview of the quality of cost of psychiatric services used by employees.

For thirty years prior to 1975, Firm B has employed a part-time physician and the clinic has been run with an "open-door" policy. In 1975 the firm has hired a new full-time physician whose interests and duties are in the area of occupational safety and health. Currently, efforts are being made to control employee access to the physician in order to free more of his time for occupational duties. Management hopes to reduce the number of employee visits to the physician by "strongly recommending" that employees who use the clinic for follow-up care or treatment of chronic conditions seek treatment instead from their personal physician; however, nurses are available to deal with some nonoccupational complaints.

The management representatives interviewed were skeptical of the posibility of expanding nonoccupational services in an industrial setting. Management views employee overutilization and attempts to get around the clinic's "occupational care only" policy as problems. Management is skeptical about the possibility of reducing health insurance premiums by offering nonoccupational services to employees, feeling that provision of these services might encourage excess utilization of physicians.

As a financial firm, Firm C has fewer occupational injuries than others in the sample. Two and a half years ago the firm began to offer physician's services to employees on a limited basis. Currently a physician is available twenty hours a week for preemployment and executive physician examinations and treatment of illnesses and injuries serious enough to require the attention of a physician. The physician is not an employee of Firm C: his services are leased from a local clinic. The cost of physician services is recovered by the savings on the cost of executive physical exams when done in-house.

In addition to the occupational services, Firm C permits employees to use the clinic for allergy immunization shots and innoculations required for foreign travel. The former service is justified by the savings of employee time previously lost traveling to outside clinics for this service. The latter service is offered as a convenience for employees.

The management representative of Firm C stated that the firm will probably not increase the scope of nonoccupational services offered to employees. If it could be demonstrated that delivery of such services would reduce the firm's overall health care costs, then such an expansion of services would be considered. Ultimately, however, delivery of nonoccupational services would probably be rejected as an intrusion into the employee's right to select his own physician and to determine the type and amount of medical care he receives.

The management representative of Firm D, whose clinic is classified as mixed, stated that the primary purposes of the employe health clinic are the prevention and treatment of industrial accidents and the reduction of absenteeism: the firm does not want to go into the medical business. This point was illustrated by two examples: the company immunizes for flu but not for polio, the latter being an extremely rare cause of absenteeism; if an employee injures his arm on the job, he receives x-rays at no cost; if he injures his arm playing tennis, he may use the company's facilities for x-rays, but he must pay for the service.

Despite this desire to avoid involvement in the "medical business," Firm D does provide a variety of medical services to its employees. Physical examinations are offered to employees on a voluntary basis. X-rays and laboratory services, as well as commonly used drugs, are offered to employees at cost for nonoccupational ailments. The company physician stated that employees occasionally use the clinic for nonoccupational care because of the convenience and short waiting periods. Increased liability for physician malpractice and objections of unfair competition from local doctors were seen as obstacles to future expansion of clinic services.

Firm E has by far the largest number of employees among those interviewed, but their dispersal over a large area presents many of the problems typically associated with a small industry. However, agreements with approximately 200 local physicians extend the effective range of employer-provided health services. The policy governing Firm E's clinic generally limits care to occupational services, with enough exceptions to justify classifying it as a mixed clinic. Health evaluations are given yearly to employees over age thirty-five. Employees are provided with retirement counseling services and with extensive counseling for emotional, drug, and alcohol problems.

Firm F's clinic, a comprehensive-type, fulfills a threefold role: occupational safety and health services for employees at the firm's various locations, preventive and primary care for all employees, and assistance for employees with psychological, alcohol, and drug problems. Preventive services include physical examinations performed regularly, the frequency increasing with employee age. According to the spokesman, every employee gets the same exam regardless of his position in the firm: there are no "executive physicals" given. Primary care is offered by means of a daily "sick call," during which employees can receive treatment for whatever complaints they present. All patients reporting to sick call are seen by a physician. The three nurses assist the physician but do not function as nurse practitioners. They do take care of minor injuries and give out aspirin, cold pills, and so on when the physician is not available.

Althought the clinic is not justified primarily in economic terms, a long-term study has been conducted by the firm of the cost of maintaining its own laboratory and x-ray department. Cost savings were found which resulted from savings in employee time that would otherwise have been spent traveling to external medical facilities. Analyses have also shown the alcoholism rehabilitation program to be cost-effective. In addition, the number of absences and accidents is decreased since the institution of safety and absentee programs.

Firm G, with approximately 6,000 employees, has the greatest involvement in nonoccupational health care of those studied. Visits total 55,000 per year to the firm's two health clinics, an average of 9.66 visits per employee. The spokesman described the services offered as "total health care" and estimated that 75 percent of the employees use the clinics as their sole source of primary care. The larger clinic has been in operation since the early 1950s, with the number of visits and the level of services remaining relatively stable over this period.

Sixteen physicians are employed by Firm G, five full-time and the remainder a half-day per week. The majority of the part-time physicians are specialists. The clinic system of using part-time specialists ensures that employees are treated by competent cost-effective physicians and controls costs of secondary care by allowing adjustment of specialist availability to employee demand. In addition to registered nurses, the clinic also employs two nurse practitioners, who handle many of the routine clinic visits.

At Firm G the clinic is viewed primarily as an employee fringe benefit, rather than a cost control mechanism. However, two studies have suggested that the clinic does justify itself in economic terms. Unfortunately, efforts to assess its effect on health insurance premiums have been thwarted by lack of data.

These seven clinics vary greatly in their physical facilities, their levels of staffing, and the range of services they provide. In part, these variations can be attributed to differences in company size and industry type. The Conference Board's survey of company health programs determined that in general a company's involvement in health care, as expressed in the number of physicians hired and its per employee investment, correlates with industry type and company size. All other factors equal, manufacturing firms and those with large employee populations are more likely to be heavily involved.[3]

Although these trends can be observed in the clinics studied, the size and the scope of health care programs in some cases vary independently of company size and industry type. For example, firms B and G are both involved in manufacturing and have a comparable number of employees, but Firm B limits its program to the delivery of occupational care while Firm G offers comprehensive services. Variations of this kind reflect each firm's conscious intent to determine the scope of its health care program, which reflects in turn its view of the purpose of the program and the resources available for it.

The management of firms that have established clinics of the occupational type (Firms A, B, and C) subscribe to the principle that the firm's primary obligation is to attempt to provent and to treat occupational injuries and illnesses. In addition, these clinics offer services seen as beneficial to the employee and the firm, but they have a narrower definition of mutual benefit than the two other types. Generally, mutual benefit is seen as a reduction in employee absenteeism. The best example of a procedure that is mutually beneficial in this sense is the treatment of minor illnesses that occur when the employee is at work. The employee benefits from free medical attention, and the employer benefits because of the short time needed to seek treatment. Flu innoculations and hypertension screening programs are mutually beneficial in the same manner.

In keeping with the limited scope of their goals, the hours of physician availability in occupational-type clinics are relatively limited. Total physician hours per month in firms A, B, and C respectively are 23 (excluding psychiatric hours), 172, and 86 (see table 2). The scheduling of physician time is dictated primarily be the volume of physical exams and other predictable services (in the case of Firm B, occupational health and safety services). Hence, management discourages employees' use of the company physician as a substitute for private physicians, However, in the firms visited, the company nurse provides some routine care and is not as strictly limited to occupational complaints as are physicians.

These firms see nursing care as an integral part of their health care programs, and in Firms A and C have recently reexamined the nurse's respon-

Table 2.
Clinic Staffing Patterns.

Firm	Physicians	Nurses	Ancillary (medical)	Specialties
A	3 part-time	1 full-time	—	general practice surgery psychiatry
B	1 full-time	4 full-time	—	surgery
C	contracts with outside clinic for physician services	3 full-time (main clinic)	—	internal medicine
D	1 full-time	3 full-time	—	internal medicine
E	3 full-time 2 part-time (20 hrs./wk.) 10 part-time (half day/wk.)		2 x-ray technicians 2 lab technicians 3 rehabilitation counselors	internal medicine radiology surgery family practice orthopedics dermatology obstetrics/gynecology
F	1 full-time	3 full-time	2 rehabilitation counselors 1 lab technician	internal medicine surgery public health
G	5 full-time 3 part-time	8 full-time [a]	1 rehabilitation counselor 2.5 full-time lab and x-ray technicians	internal medicine surgery endocrinology hematology allergy dermatology

[a]Includes two nurse practitioners.

sibilities. Firm A has expanded the role of the company nurse to encompass occupational safety and health education. This change was motivated by dissatisfaction with the traditional role of the nurse in the occupational clinic, which has often been limited to providing temporary care for minor illnesses and injuries. The nurse at Firm A still provides the traditional services, but her duties have been expanded in the hope of increasing her impact on employee health. At Firm C, management expressed a similar desire to upgrade nursing care and is currently subsidizing the further education of the clinic nurse for the purpose of introducing nurse practitioners into their clinics. They hope to enhance the quality of care while maintaining the current scope of clinic services. Firm C shares this desire to maintain its current level of services with other occupational clinics in the sample. An advantage of the occupational-type clinic is that its scope of care is clearly defined. Employees are expected to cooperate and use the clinic exclusively for occupational ailments. Expansion of clinic services will be encouraged only if the benefits can be demonstrated to be greater than the costs resulting from expanding beyond these clearly defined boundaries.

The services offered in the mixed-type clinics surveyed (Firms D and E), resemble to an extent those of the occupational clinics. Mixed clinic exceptions to an "occupational care only" policy, however, permit clinic personnel to provide a significant amount of nonoccupational health services. Nonetheless, the health care programs of Firms D and E differ widely in philosophy. In Firm D, primary care services are offered on a drop-in basis. Treatment of employees is at the discretion of the physician, and nurses free his time by treating many of the routine cases. Firm D's physician can be seen as an extension of the employee's personal physician, providing much the same services when it is inconvenient for the employee to see his personal physician. In contrast, Firm E's nonoccupational services are almost exclusively diagnostic or preventive. Its periodic health evaluation and retirement counseling services are seen as first steps in an effort to create a preventive care and health care management program. This program is not intended as an additional source of primary care for employees, but rather as a new kind of service that supplements and integrates the care provided by physicians.

Firms D and E differ greatly in size and in the geographic distribution of their employee populations, and each health care program fits the firm's particular situation. Firm D's clinic serves a large, concentrated employee population and can offer limited primary care services as a benefit to employees without distracting the physician from his primary function, the treatment and prevention of industrial accidents. Firm E, on the other hand, has a large and highly dispersed employee population. Primary care services could be provided as a secondary benefit only at locations where sufficient concentrations of employees exist to justify hiring a physician for occupational safety and health needs, leaving other employees without access to services. However, this firm's preventive health and health care management approach generates visits that are more predictable and easily scheduled, permits equal access for all employees, and has the advantage of limiting the number of visits. Visits average about 1 per employee-year, as opposed to 3.10 at Firm D and, to contrast a comprehensive program, 9.66 at Firm G. The contrasting approaches of Firm D and E to employee health care suggest that differences in corporate mission and geographic distribution of employees have a great deal to do with determining the orientation of clinics that offer more than traditional services.

The wide range of nonoccupational health services offered by the comprehensive-type clinics early distinguishes them from clinics in the occupational and mixed categories. The health care programs of Firms F and G contain three elements: occupational health and safety services, nonoccupational care (including primary care and preventive services), and employee counseling. Physicians in the two firms reported that the clinics were the sole source of primary care for a portion of the employees, estimated at 75 percent in Firm G. In addition, both firms have organized counseling programs for employees with emotional, alcohol, or drug problems. Spokesmen for both firms stressed, however, that occupational safety and health are major priorities in their clinic programs.

Firms F and G justify their additional services primarily in noneconomic terms: they are viewed primarily as employee fringe benefits. Both firms report, however, that their clinic programs are cost-effective. Careful staff selection ensures that employees will be treated by high qualitv physicians (the majority of physicians on the staff at Firms F and G have faculty appointments at area medical schools). Firm F, as previously noted, has performed cost studies over long periods of time that demonstrate that x-ray and laboratory services justify themselves financially in terms of employee time saved by not traveling for these services. Firm G also claims that staffing their clinic with a variety of part-time specialists yields some measure of cost control. Finally, both firms feel that the comprehensive clinic program improves the overall health status of their employee populations and results in less frequent use of services from outside providers. Both firms see these factors as helping to keep growing health insurance premiums under control, although they admit that this kind of effect is particularly difficult to demonstrate.

Despite similar program goals and levels of service, two significant differences can be found in the staffing patterns of these clinics. In Firm F, the majority of employees who visit the clinic (estimated at 50 to 60 percent) are seen by a physician, while Firm G uses nurses, including two nurse practitioners, for routine procedures. The two programs also differ in their use of specialists. Overall, Firm F has the fewer physicians, owing at least in part to the greater dispersal of its employees.

The variations in staffing patterns take on significance when it is recalled that a good portion of industry's expenditures for health care represents the salaries of physicians and nurses. Although there is much diversity among the sample in clinic staffing, the strategies of Firm F and G illustrate two basic approaches used by all the firms. Firms A, B, C, and D use (although to varying extents) what could be termed a screening strategy: nurses handle routine visits, freeing the physician to handle the more complex cases and other duties. In Firms E and F, on the other hand, the majority of patients see the physician. Although the roles of nurse practitioners have not been firmly delineated, their potential for rendering quality care at lower costs for certain procedures is generally accepted. The large number of visits to some of the clinics (see table

3) suggests that many are made because of the convenience of the clinic and the complaints would be self-treated if the clinic were not available. The United States average is 4.9 visits to the physicians' office per employee-year in metropolitan areas with populations under 1,000,000.[4] The immediate problem at clinics with such high utilization rate is screening the minor cases out from the more serious. Nurse practitioners might prove a cost-effective solution to this problem.

The decision whether to use specialist versus generalist physicians in the industrial clinic is more complex, but an important one in providing comprehensive care. Secondary care is in general more expensive, but there may be advantages to making specialists available to employees if complicated medical problems are to be cared for. In order to provide general guidelines for the use of specialists in industrial clinics, much currently inaccessible data will be needed.

The clinic policies and programs reviewed here have implications both for health care delivery and for health professional training programs, corporate as well as for the delivery system as a whole. The occupational-type clinic represents the traditional approach to the problems of worker health. Physicians staffing these clinics have expertise in occupational health and safety, grounded in a knowledge of toxology and emergency medicine. In keeping with the policy of the firm, the physician has limited involvement in the workers' nonoccupational health care. The operating principles of the mixed and comprehensive clinics, on the other hand, are based on the premise that

Table 3.
Clinic Utilization and Cost per Visit, 1976.

Firm	Number Employed	Annual Visits (all facilities)	Visits per Employee	Cost per Visit
A	600	5,250[a]	8.75	N/A[b]
B[c]	4,000	22,000[d]	5.5	N/A
C[e]	5,400	19,184	3.55	$8.48
D	4,000	12,532	3.10	N/A
E	30,000	30,000	1	$26.66
F	4,000	N/A	N/A	N/A
G	6,000	55,000	9.66	$12.50[f]

[a]Based on estimate by plant nurse of 10–15 patients per day; does not include informal visits outside clinic.
[b]Not available.
[c]Based on figures collected before change in clinic policy.
[d]1974.
[e]Includes employees on visits from smaller branch facility.
[f]Cost in largest facility; smaller facility slightly lower.

benefits can be gained by having nonoccupational medical services provided by health professionals who are familiar with both the worker and workplace.

The conviction that the industrial physician should provide nonoccupational care has given rise to two models of industrial health care. In one model (illustrated in this sample by Firm E and presented in chapter 2 by Collings), the industrial physician functions as a health care manager. Using periodic health evaluations and epidemiological expertise, he works with the patient's personal physician to supplement and integrate the care provided by the prvate sector. The other model (illustrated by Firms F, and G, and to a lesser extend D, and presented in chapter 5 by Greer, et al.), is based on the assumption that high quality, cost-effective care can be provided when the company physician functions as the worker's primary care physician. The evidence suggests that both these approaches may be valid, depending on patterns of employee dispersal. It seems quite likely that they will coexist in the future.

It is clear, furthermore, that a variety of types of industrial clinics currently exist. This finding has great significance for those who train "industrial physicians." Should the industrial physicians of the future be trained strictly as occupational health physicians, or should managerial and primary care skills also be emphasized? Should three types of industrial physicians be trained: a physician-manager, an occupational safety and health physician, and an industrial primary care physician? Or is it possible for a physician to be adequately trained in all three areas without conflict?

Similar questions can be posed regarding the role of the industrial clinic in the health care delivery system. Can the industrial clinic be integrated into the overall system? Or will expanding industrial clinics bring on further fragmentation of the health care delivery system? It is possible that comprehensive-type clinics can serve as a focus for a new form of hybrid prepaid health plan for employees and their families, on the experience of Firm G.[5] Only time will provide the answers to these questions, but industry has such a large stake in the control of health care costs that surely attempts will be made to maximize the potential of industrial health clinics.

NOTES

1. Duan Block, "Postgraduate Training of the Occupational Physician," *Journal of the American Occupational Medical Association*, November 1976, pp. 755–766.

2. Seymour Lusterman, *Industry Roles in Health Care* (New York: The Conference Board, 1974); and *The Complex Puzzle of Rising Health Care Costs: Can the Private Sector Fit It Together?* (Washington, D.C.: President's Council on Wage and Price Stability, 1976).

3. Lusterman, op. cit., p. 29.

4. U.S. Department of Health, Education, and Welfare, Public Health Service, *Forward Plan for Health, FY 1978–1982* (Washtington, D.C., 1976).

5. Richard H. Egdahl and Diana Chapman Walsh, "Industry-Sponsored Health Programs: A New Hybrid Prepaid Plan," *New England Journal of Medicine*, 296:1350–1353, 1977.

Corporate Mental Health Benefits*

Willis B. Goldbeck

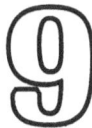

Public understanding and professional treatment of mental illness has a history of which we can only be embarrassed. For reasons steeped in myth, fear, confusion, and ignorance, illness of the mind has frequently been viewed as a category of disease separate from that affecting any other part of the human body. It is all right to break an arm, have a kidney fail, succumb courageously to cancer, or use the ears and nose to support a strange apparatus designed to assist our eyes. But the mind, that is different. That we were all supposed to totally control—by ourselves. And, if something should be a bit abnormal, therapy often entails more ostracism than rehabilitation. With such a history, it is little wonder that the evolution of employee health benefits offered coverage for nearly every other human organ and disease before including the mind and its problems.

Mental illness is treated more openly now. Even the lingering presence of

*This paper and the survey upon which it is based were prepared with the appreciated assistance of Saul Kilstein and Andy Weinberg . . . and seventy-nine corporate leaders.

the Willowbrookes (New York City) and St. Elizabeth's (Washington, D.C.) serves to remind us more of the horrors that used to be than of today's promise. Many factors have contributed to this slow change. Psychiatry became popularized through its use by public idols. New drugs produced a new era in therapy. The mass media first sensationalized and then helped legitimize the severity of mental illness' negative impact on society as a whole. We became, especially in the 1960s, increasingly aware that narcotics, alcoholism, and sexual dysfunction were not just "problems," but actual, treatable illnesses. As the sphere of acknowledged mental illness expanded beyond that of mental retardation, a greater proportion of the population was encompassed. And, even if it did not include us, we all knew someone who. . . .

In effect, mental illness had to be popularized before it could become recognized for what it really is. Even the medical profession contributed to the confusion. For decades, physicians have known that a significant proportion of the physical ailments they were asked to cure were actually the manifestations of mental problems they were ill-equipped to treat. Patients, however, do not want *not* to be treated, and the reimbursement system has never rewarded physicians for not treating, so it is easy to see the pressures that have kept mental illness in the proverbial closet.

Today, there are new pressures—and new evidence of the relationship between mental illness and physical symptoms. And, like everything else in the health care area, the total cost of care is one of the major stimulants for taking a new look at mental health. If treating mental health problems can be shown to reduce the overall rate of health care cost escalation, that—more than any scientific, medical, or humanitarian breakthrough—will make such treatment publicly acceptable.

Previously, there existed no single source to which one could turn for a concise review of the mental health segment of major corporate health benefit programs. In an effort to overcome this, report on current trends, and begin to measure the impact of employee mental health benefits, we at the Washington Business Group on Health are conducting a survey of our 145 members (see exhibit 1). Later, this will be expanded with a revised questionnaire to include many other large employers. This report is based upon the first 79 replies.

All 79 of the respondents provide a program of mental health benefits. Naturally, the coverage, administration, and financing vary, but many commonalities do exist and certain generalizations can be drawn. The major findings relating to the extent of coverage are: mental health benefits are equally available to all employees (96%). The benefits are extended to dependents (between 61% and 90%, depending on the benefit) and to retirees (37%–67%). Schizophrenia, depression, and alcohol and drug dependencies are the disorders most commonly covered (71%–90%). However, Family-marital-sexual problems are just beginning to be included as a covered benefit (less than 25%).

Survey findings relating to financing are: only 1 of the 79 corporations uses a prepaid program. Blue Cross–Blue Shield (33%) and the commercial carriers (72%) account for all the plans, including cases of coverage divided among more than one class of carrier. Many companies insure their plans with several commercial carriers, with the Equitable, Metropolitan, and Travelers the most frequently named. There is an almost even split between those companies that pay 100% of the premium for the mental health benefit (52%) and those that share the cost with the employees (48%). For those that share, the employee's portion is most commonly limited to 20 percent or less. The preference for providing benefits through insurance rather than through the direct provision of care can be seen in table 1.

Each company was asked to identify the ways it felt the provision of mental health benefits helped the company:

Improved employee moral	52%
Lowered employee absenteeism	53%
Fewer instances of *severe* mental illness	51%
Improved employee productivity	53%
Reduced hospital utilization	46%
Lower total insurance premiums	16%

It would be impossible to look at this list and not notice two things: the motivation rarely lies in simply "saving money," and there is an apparent inconsistency in that 51 percent expect to reduce incidents of severe mental illness and 46 percent expect to see a reduction in hospital utilization, yet only 16 percent expect to see a reduction in total insurance premiums.

The companies were asked, "Which of the following constraints have employers with in-house mental health programs encountered?" The survey replies did not provide an exact count of in-house programs. The list and percentages that follow are based upon the thirty-two companies that provided a clear description of their in-house program.

Identifying employees in need of assistance	66%
Removing stigmas associated with treatment of mental illness	53%
Training supervisors to detect mental illness and make necessary referrals (but avoiding "witch hunts")	41%
Developing a company policy on confidentiality	34%
Motivating employees to obtain treatment	50%
Assuring no negative consequences to employment status for those who do obtain treatment	25%

It is of particular interest, we feel, that the constraint that received the least response was the one about negative employment consequences. One can only hope that the proportion would be the same were the survey responded to by the employees.

It is common knowledge that the incentives provided by our traditional

Exhibit 1
Washington Business Group on Health

AMAX	Corning Glass Works
AMF	Deere & Company
ASARCO	Deering Milliken
Aetna	Dow Chemical, USA
Allis Chalmers	Dresser
Alcoa	E. I. duPont
American Can	Eastman Kodak
American Cyanamid	Eaton
American Medical International	Eli Lilly
AT&T	Equitable Life
Armco Steel	Esmark
Armstrong Cork	Exxon
Atlantic Richfield	FMC
Babcock & Wilcox	Federated Department Stores
Becton, Dickinson & Company	Firestone
Bethlehem Steel	Ford
Boeing	General Electric
Boise Cascade	General Foods
Bristol Myers	General Mills
George B. Buck	General Motors
Budd	GTE
Burlington Industries	General Tire & Rubber
Burlington Northern	GENESCO
Campbell Soup	Georgia-Pacific
Carter Hawley Hale	B. F. Goodrich
Caterpillar Tractor	Goodyear
Chrysler	Greyhound
Citibank	Gulf Oil
Cities Service	Hanna Mining
Clark Equipment	Harris Trust & Savings
Coca-Cola	Heinz, USA
Columbia Gas	C. T. Hellmut & Associates
Connecticut General	Hercules
Continental Bank	Honeywell
Continental Group	Inland Steel
Continental Oil	Inmont Corporation
Coopers & Lybrand	IBM

Exhibit 1
Washington Business Group on Health

International Harvester
Jewel Companies
John Hancock
Johns-Manville
Jones & Laughlin Steel
Kaiser
Kennecott Copper
Koppers
LTV
Libbey-Owens-Ford
3M
Marathon Oil
Marcor
Martin Marietta
Mead
Merck
Metropolitan Life
Mobil Oil
Monsanto
National Steel
Northern Natural Gas
Olin
Owens-Corning Fiberglas
Owens-Illinois
PPG Industries
Pet
Pfizer
Philip Morris
Pitney Bowes
Procter & Gamble
Prudential
Pullman
RCA
R. J. Reynolds Industries
Ralston Purina
Republic Steel
Reynolds Metals

Rockwell International
SCM
St. Regis Paper
Scott Paper
Sears, Roebuck
Shell Oil
Sherwin-Williams
Singer
A. O. Smith
SmithKline
Southern California Edison
Sperry Rand
Standard Oil of California
Standard Oil (Indiana)
Stanley Works
Stauffer Chemical
Sun Company
Sundstrand Chemical
TRW
Tenneco
Texaco
Texas Gas Transmission
Texas Instruments
Travelers
Union Camp
Union Carbide
Union Electric
Union Pacific
Uniroyal
U.S. Steel
Westinghouse Electric
Weyerhaeuser
Whirlpool
Xerox

Table 1.
Means of Providing Mental Health Care.

Benefit	Corporate Medical Department	Independent Contractor	Insurance Benefit
Psychiatric care	8	8	67
Alcohol disorders	22	8	58
Drug dependencies	19	6	54

reimbursement system, combined with benefit designs that have encouraged the use of the most expensive facilities and treatment procedures, have contributed greatly to rampant cost escalation. We asked a series of questions seeking to determine whether the same problems were being built into the mental health benefits. The results are mixed. Most (75%) replied that they do not provide incentives that "encourage early detection and treatment." However, 49 percent do allow charges for treatment in an inpatient facility "other than a hospital," and, even more importantly, 78 of the 79 now cover charges of a physican for psychiatric treatment in outpatient settings. However, these benefits typically carry a 20–50 percent copayment and some also involve a small deductible. Also, 63 percent allow charges by a physician or hospital for psychiatric treatment under "in residence" programs when the patient may be allowed to go home at night or to work during the day in order to prevent complete severance from a natural environment. Further, 80 percent provide reimbursements for mental health practitioners other than physicians. Specifically mentioned were:

Psychologists: few limitations; some require physician direction or supervision; generally same as psychiatrists;

Social workers: less frequently accepted; often limited to team work in a "recognized" facility;

Psychiatric nurses: not common; where accepted, the limits are generally the same as for other RNs.

We found that very few (12%) of the companies had a measurable decrease in "visits to physicians for nonmedical reasons owing to the provision of mental health benefits." However, since another 34 percent had not even attempted such a measurement, these results are far from conclusive.

Data on the cost of mental health benefits are scarce. Only 32 percent of the respondents were able to provide any information, and several of these could provide only estimates. It is important to note that, with only one or two exceptions, the lack of response does not imply a lack of willingness to open their books. In fact, the problem exists for the best of reasons: most companies have not segregated their costs by disease, and they now view mental illness as just another disease.

From those that did respond, some rough averages can be shown. Approximately 5 percent of total health benefits costs can be attributed to mental health benefits or service. The monthly per capita premium for mental health benefits has a broad range: $4.35 to $78.00. The average is $29.47.

Some of the companies have gone beyond the normal insured medical benefits program. General Foods is a good example. Their insured medical plan is described in a brochure for employees:

> When an employee or dependent is hospitalized for treatment of a mental or nervous condition, benefits are paid just as for any other confinement. There is no deductible, no coinsurance, and benefits are paid in semiprivate accommodations for up to 365 days.

> When an employee or dependent receives nonhospital treatment for a mental/nervous condition—for example, visits to a psychiatrist's office— these are considered Class B benefits and paid at 50% after the $75 individual deductible; there is a family deductible of $150.

In addition, the company offers a Troubled Employee Assistance Program. The program is described:

> The company offers confidential help and the opportunity of rehabilitation to employees who may be troubled by alcoholism, drug abuse, mental illness, or emotional disturbances caused by family and financial problems. Any of the problems can have a serious effect on an individual's personal life and job performance.

An introductory statement by General Foods' chairman sets the tone that is essential for employee acceptance:

> It is estimated that as many as 15 million working Americans may be troubled by alcoholism, drug abuse, mental illness, or emotional problems caused by family or financial problems. These illnesses strike at all organizational levels in industry. No one is really immune. Fortunately, if illnesses of this kind are detected and treated at an early stage, they can usually be overcome.

> General Foods, where you spend almost a third of your life, is concerned about these illnesses and wants to help its troubled employees. Help will be given professionally, confidentially, and with full respect for the dignity of the individual.

Corporate mental health benefits and programs are not *the* solution to the health care cost problem, nor are they *the* answer to decades of ill-informed neglect of mental illness. Nonetheless, the efforts of employers, often with union cooperation, are making millions of Americans aware that mental illness is just as normal, or no more abnormal, than any physical dysfunction. The trends are clear: more insured mental health benefits and an increasing number of companies offering direct counseling and other services through their own medical facilities. Although the survey did not indicate this, private conversations lead us to believe that there will soon be substantial movement toward the provision of mental health benefits on a prepaid basis.

Further, we feel that the survey shows that there is much less problem with confidentiality and fear of job loss than is commonly expressed. There are many reasons for this, not the least of which has been union insistance upon safeguards, but the fact remains that most employers can see the value of a well-designed mental health benefits program and know that it cannot succeed without the full confidence of the employees. Finally, as employers become more aggressively, and directly, involved in the provision of medical care, they will become an increasingly significant force for positive change in the treatment of mental illness.

Foundations for Medical Care and Corporate Health Benefits

George Himler

10

Any self-respecting analyst of the American health care system is constrained to begin with a gloomy statement on the high costs of medical services. Since custom also dictates a little hyperbole, it becomes mandatory for him to use such descriptions as "escalating," "soaring," "skyrocketing," and "relentless inflation." Finally, no presentation can be considered complete unless it includes an extrapolation of the rate of cost increases, with or without graph, which leads to the inevitable conclusion that by the year 2000, unless the author's favorite remedy is applied, expenditures for health services will exceed the GNP by 50 percent. This analyst has neither the courage nor the inclination to flout tradition, so let us consider that the dire statements and predictions have all been made and get on with some history, some diagnosis, and some suggestions for therapy.

After World War II medicine in the United States entered a halcyon period of growing demand, increasing public expectations, and almost unlimited funding. Research was supported by government with little discrimination as to its nature, cost, and probable usefulness. A need was perceived to modernize existing facilities and build new ones, and the Hill-Burton program led to a veritable binge of hospital construction. Sophisticated and expensive equipment was acquired by institutions almost haphazardly, without regard to its utilization or areawide distribution.

At the same time, the various insurance and funding mechanisms, culminating in the open-ended Medicare and Medicaid programs, accommodated progressive increases in total professional fees and institutional reimbursement. With government subsidies, medical school output was expanded in a decade from approximately 9,000 to more than 16,000 graduates per year. The philosophy that "more is better" flourished unchecked. As recently as the late 1960s, health economists and other public health types were still loudly proclaiming shortages of human and physical health care resources.

It is unhappy but true that monumental binges are followed by equally monumental hangovers. Health care is no exception. Although the signs were there before, it was not until the early 1970s that it became unmistakably clear that Medicare and Medicaid were totally out of control. At about the same time, the Blue Cross and Blue Shield plans, particularly the former, began to line up regularly at insurance commissioners' doors for rate increases, which were usually granted, amid howls of public indignation. Other health and hospital insurance carriers followed suit. Those who paid insurance premiums out of their own pockets felt the increases most immediately and were badly hurt. The rate increments affected union and employer health benefits as well, giving rise to a crescendo of discomfort and alarm in those quarters that still shows no signs of peaking out.

Suddenly, everyone was perceiving excesses where there had been only shortages before. We are now told that our hospital system is approximately 20 percent "overbedded." Hospitals have duplicates of expensive equipment and services that are underutilized. We have an excessive number of physicians and specialists in relation to the population. The utilization of beds and services is out of sight. Unit costs are unbearable. Medical school subsidies are too high. Research support is excessive and the research itself is uncoordinated. And on and on.

Undismayed by having to do an about-face, the health analysts, economists, administrators, and legislators adopted a new credo and have apparently rationalized it to their own satisfaction. These modern disciples of Procrustes, who, until recently, were busy advocating S–T–R–E–T–C–H–I–N–G the capacity of the health care delivery system, are now equally engrossed in devising methods of chopping off parts they deem excessive or unnecessary. Thus we are treated to a barrage of well-intentioned, heroic, and almost certainly self-defeating recommendations and practices.

Typical of these measures is cutting back program benefits "across the board." Another is the imposition of "caps" on cost increases or total expenditures. A third favorite expedient is reimbursing for hospital services through a prospective budget based on costs that are three years or more out of date and expecting the hospitals to effect these savings without diminishing or impairing care. A final cost control idea whose time whould probably never have come is that of the so-called DRGs or diagnosis related groups, which would have hospitals paid by diagnosis, regardless of the patients' specific needs or lengths of stay. This device would go far toward guaranteeing the creation of overwhelming incentives to minimize patient care and compromise its quality.

The fundamental characteristic common to all these proposed or actual practices is that they are merely gross limits and restraints applied without judgment, discrimination, or evaluation of specific circumstances in individual institutions and regions. Similar restraints are in effect, or contemplated, for the payment of physicians and other practitioners in tax supported programs, without regard to the welfare of the programs' beneficiaries. Simultaneously, there is a loud hue and cry about fraud and abuse, although no one seems to have any idea of the magnitude of the problem or how to cope with it. All in all, an objective observer must conclude that current efforts at control and retrenchment are as frenetic, irrational, and ill-advised as were the expansionist programs of the previous decade.

It is undeniable that an annual 16 percent increment in reimbursement, particularly to hospitals and extended care facilities, is dismaying. Yet that annual rise exceeds that of the consumer price index primarily because the institutions' expenditures are heavily weighted by high-cost components such as labor and specialized supplies and equipment. It would therefore be simplistic to argue that the spending of 8 to 8.5 percent GNP on health services is unwarranted. It may or may not be, depending on how we define health care, and how we want it provided and distributed. While the gross annual cost estimates of $118 billion and $140 billion are certainly impressive, there has been no consensus on what proportion of GNP should be allotted to health care in relation to expenditures for other essential goods and services such as housing, food, energy, and transportation, to name only a few. Granted that reduction, or at least containment, of health care costs is urgent, that fact should not be used to justify the draconian measures currently being advocated or put into effect. It is obvious that this nation has been examining and evaluating its health care system for decades and that current pressures for change are not based on financial considerations alone.

Since restructuring of the delivery and payment mechanisms seems imminent, it should be a major concern of all involved that in striving for immediate economy we avoid overreacting and destroying concepts, manpower resources, institutions, and facilities that we have created over the years and that should be preserved as essential elements of an effective health system. There are nondestructive means at hand for achieving substantial reductions now, and they should be applied, but with the understanding that, unless current social and economic trends are modified or reversed, costs will inevitably resume their upward course.

Since we have not accepted, and probably will not adopt, policies to deny universal access to needed services or to subjugate quality to pure cost considerations, the major thrust must be to eliminate waste, optimize utilization, and redesign program benefits to provide alternative, and more economical, levels of treatment where appropriate. Simultaneous assessment of the quality of care will be needed to prevent deterioration of services. This would not be an easy assignment for even a single agncy with all the financial resources, data, analytic and planning skills, and authorizations that will be required. It seems almost impossible of accomplishment for the crazy-quilt body of planning authorities, programs, sponsors, administrators, and funding agencies that will be addressing themselves to it.

As far as its own programs are concerned, the federal government, in providing substantial support for health maintenance organizations (HMOS) and independent practice associations (IPAs) and by creating professional standards review organizations (PSROs), has shown some understanding of the problems, while tacitly admitting its inability to solve them administratively. The states, which have had disastrous experiences with their administration of Medicaid, have generally undertaken their own corrective measures with such little aptitude and finesse that the programs in many states are either grossly inadequate or in total disarray. Therefore, although we recognize that most initiatives for cost control and modification of health care delivery have organized in the public sector, we must look to the private sector for active leadership in the future.

The private sector should be powerfully motivated to develop and undertake its own health care programs and improve existing ones, if for no other reason than to forestall government intervention and to assure a nonpolitical, objective, rational, and moderate approach. What elements of the private sector must be involved? Industry comes to mind most immediately. Aside from its tax contributions to support federal and state programs and its direct contributions to disability and Workmen's Compensation insurance, industry supports extensive employee health benefit programs through direct premium payments or self-insurance. In spite of these massive contributions industry is virtually powerless to negotiate its costs and has no control whatever over the quality of the care its money buys. It is not suggested that industry merely lend its efforts to evolving delivery and payment systems that might be implemented at some future time. Since the development program would be based on review of the utilization of health services there would be an immediate payoff in the form of reduction or containment of current costs.

A second and more important participant in the private effort would be the insurance industry. Through the years carriers have undertaken experiments with new payment mechanisms and new modalities of health care delivery. Even now there may be forty such experimental programs in progress with a total investment by the carriers of approximately $80 million. In spite of the magnitude of the sum expended, the various programs have been uncoordinated and a number of them have failed. As a result, some carriers have abandoned the concept entirely. There are indications, however, that interest is reawakening and that many carriers are ready to resume an active role in experimentation with review methods and delivery systems to "normalize" expenditures.

Since the insurance industry has been widely criticized for failing to have programs for utilization and cost control in effect, it too would derive an immediate benefit from the application of functioning review programs to its insured population. Such involvement on the part of the carriers would help contain premium increases and relieve carriers of the onus of being indifferent to cost control as long as their premiums are increased regularly.

The final key group will be the health professionals, particularly physicians. Since the bulk of medical services is delivered by physicians practicing individually or in small groups, doctors have been difficult or impossible to reach for purposes of health care planning, let alone direct negotiations. Their medical societies and specialty associations were not designed to serve these functions, nor are they authorized to commit their physician members to anything except very broad policy. In the past, only the members of the old-line medical care foundations (FMCs) and closed-panel groups were approachable in this sense. More recently, with renewed interest and funding for HMOs operating in conjunction with IPAs, physicians are again beginning to organize along medical care foundation lines. Through these organizations and through PSROs, which enjoy very substantial physician membership and good relations with the other health professions, physicians can participate actively in the planning and implementation of new programs.

The FMCs, HMO/IPAs, and PSROs can and do relate to local industry and to the carriers that function in their own areas. Such local involvement is excellent but if national employers and carriers are to be involved in review and in devising alternate delivery systems, as they must be, they must have a single organization to talk to and negotiate with. This contingency was anticipated some time ago. The American Association of Foundations for Medical Care (AAFMC) was established in 1967 to coordinate the activities of FMCs, represent them nationally, and give them technical advice and support. It presently has a membership of seventy organizations.

In 1973, the AAFMC recognized that PSROs would be in need of a similar national organization and formed the American Association of Professional Service Review Organizations (AAPSRO), first as a subsidiary and subsequently as an affiliate that is now almost autonomous. Through PSROs and FMCs, a rather large percentage of the independently practicing physicians and small group practitioners of this nation can now be involved in review programs. Furthermore, through AAFMC and its constituent foundations and HMO/IPAs, they can participate in group negotiations and health care delivery without making a quantum leap from individual to group practice.

What, then, is the next step? To begin with, the three groups must initiate a dialogue to identify problems and assess their resources. They must determine the levels at which they will function and the manner in which they can coordinate their planning and their programs. The AAFMC and AAPSRO, as the national organizations representing FMCs and PSROs, have already begun that dialogue with some employers, carriers, and carrier organizations. As a result of their utilization review experience, they have been able to give the employers and carriers some insight into the nature and dimensions of their problems, and suggestions for some preliminary solutions.

At this point, as a quick review of those problems, it is appropriate to examine abuse, utilization, and program benefits in somewhat greater detail. There are unquestionably major abuses in public programs, such as Medicare and Medicaid, in terms of kickbacks and fraudulent billing. There are also abusive practices on the part of practitioners and suppliers, such as rendering unnecessary services and overbilling. If these conditions prevail in public programs, they probably exist in private programs as well. For the purposes of control and cost reduction, therefore, and in the interest of justice, outright abuse and fraud must be eliminated. However, there is some question as to the magnitude of the problem as far as the actual dollar impact is concerned.

There is a second, more prevalent, more subtle, and probably more important type of overutilization, which is misuse. Patients and physicians alike are one step removed from the funding of health care. On the patient's part, once he has paid his premium, or it has been paid for him, he has no interest whatever in limiting the services he utilizes. Indeed, he tends to resent any restriction on his benefits and, if experience with automobile and other types of liability insurance is any criterion, he will do what he can to "beat the system." Thus we have the extra visit to the emergency room or the doctor's office and the extra day or two of hospitalization for convenience, which our public morality does not recognize as fraudulent. Nevertheless, while the individual instances of misuse do not usually involve startling amounts of money, the cumulative cost effect can be staggering.

In turn, physicians who authorize the use of services and who therefore in a sense control utilization, are not trained, conditioned, or motivated to be thrifty with program funds. They tend to overutilize services and facilities partly to benefit their patients, partly for their own convenience, and partly as a defense against malpractice litigation. The important point, however, is that they have no positive incentive to be good managers of the funds of health care plans in which they have no involvement.

A third, and extremely costly type of misuse arises from the structure of the benefit packages themselves. I is common, for instance, that certain services are reimbursable if the patient is hospitalized but not if he receives the same care in an ambulatory setting. To spare the patient out-of-pocket expense, many services are rendered in hospitals that could be done just as well on an ambulatory basis. Since this adds the cost of the most expensive facility to that of the service, it imposes a tremendous additional burden on the program. This practice could be virtually eliminated by the provision of parallel coverage in the benefit packages.

Finally, the availability of alternate levels of care is also an important factor. When a patient no longer requires acute hospital care but cannot be discharged to self care, he normally is transferred to another, less expensive institution that can provide him with the less sophisticated services he requires. If that transfer cannot be made for lack of a bed in an appropriate facility, he is retained in the acute care hospital as long as necessary, and at considerable extra cost.

In the light of these observations and experiences, the first recommendation that AAFMC and AAPSRO made to employers and the insurance industry was that they institute utilization review in their program using experienced local review organizations. At the same time, it was recognized that employers and carriers of national and regional scope could not readily negotiate for review with large numbers of local agencies which could be either FMCs or PSROs. Furthermore, the directors of the two organizations identified a need for the evaluation and certification of each review agency's capabilities and an ongoing monitoring of the review it undertakes. It was obvious that if a broad-based review program was to be undertaken by industry, those and other functions would have to be centralized. Accordingly, the boards of the AAFMC and AAPSRO authorized the incorporation of another organization known as the Peer Review Network (PRN). This is an independent, not-for-profit corporation chartered in the District of Columbia with a board of directors composed of directors of the two parent organizations. For purposes of review only, PRN will be the agency through which major employers and carriers, who operate multistate and national programs, will relate to local review agencies. Representing as it does those member organizations of AAFMC and AAPSRO that wish to participate in network review, PRN constitutes the only viable, functioning, and effective review system that can claim anything approaching national distribution. That nationwide network is now in place. It is admittedly not yet complete in its coverage, there is some variation among the local review organizations in the efficacy of their systems, and review is still concentrated on acute hospital care. Nevertheless, it is a system in being, it is being expanded actively, and it has a massive store of experience to draw on—improved standards of performance are being met.

What can employers can the insurance industry expect of utilization review and medical care evaluation? Ideally, these related but distinct activities are based on professionally developed norms, standards, and criteria and are carried out under medical control. They have a number of outcomes that are of value to patients and the financers of care. To begin with, the mere knowledge that a review system is operative has a salutary deterrent effect on individuals who habitually abuse or misuse the program. Moreover, the system identifies specific instances of inappropriate utilization or poor care and minimizes their future occurrence through physician and patient education, denials of payment, sanctions, or all three. The process creates a data base for provider, practitioner, and patient profiles, which individually serve to focus review on areas that are likely to be most productive. The same data and profiles, disidentified and combined, yield aggregate statistical data that are invaluable in areawide planning. Finally, and perhaps most importantly, the data will suggest what alternate care facilities and services should be developed and how benefit structures could be modified to take advantage of the new "mix," thereby reducing costs.

Some of the benefits of review are therefore immediate, some, more remote, but all are important—a fact that is not universally recognized. Legislators, administrators, and some professionals who are antagonistic to the review concept have raised a question as to the cost-effectiveness of utilization review. Experience in Denver and Portland has shown that proper review can save approximately eight times what it costs. An analysis of more extensive review by PSROs should yield further hard data on cost-effectiveness in the course of the next year or two.

The in-hospital review process is not cheap, however, the national range being $12 to $16 per admission. Furthermore, as the application of concurrent review approaches its objective of normalizing utilization, its cost-effectiveness will decline in proportion to the success it achieves. It should be borne in mind, however, that when this happens, a portion of the resources and personnel devoted to in-hospital review can be shifted to the review of patients across the board and care delivered in other settings. It is not the intent that each service and each encounter be reviewed ad infinitum. The system itself will be refined, improved, and expanded to accept and process data from all sources and minimize costly individual review. It is reasonable to conclude, therefore, that utilization review is cost-effective now and will remain so in the foreseeable future.

If this is true, it would be logical to ask why we need to look further for solutions to the problem of rising costs than review and the control measures that arise from it. The answer, quite simply, is that surveillance and externally imposed controls are not ideal in that they must be continuous to be effective. Furthermore, they give rise to a state of mind that invites resistance and evasion. In theory, and in practice, it is preferable to modify physician and patient behavior patterns by giving them incentives to be frugal in their use of the health care dollar. A degree of behavior modification can be achieved through education but financial incentives usually work better. Patients, for instance, might be given rebates or reduced premiums based on utilization. The rebates and reductions, of course, would be of a magnitude to create incentive and still not constitute experience rating.

Physicians' behavior and motivation can be altered by making them participants and partners in the delivery system, rather than individual entrepreneurs who merely look to benefit programs for payment and to their patients for supplementation. The mechanism for doing this was the salient feature of the early FMCs, and has been adopted, with variations, by more recently established FMCs and HMO/IPAs. It consists of putting the participating physicians of a program "at risk," thereby making them partial underwriters of the losses that may be incurred in any contract period. The basic concept is that the FMC or HMO contracts for the care of a patient group at a fixed rate for a specified period. The scope of benefits is defined, but there is usually no limit on frequency of services. Physicians are recruited from the area, who agree to treat plan patients in their own offices and in hospitals on a fee-for-service basis, using either a fixed fee schedule or the usual, customary, and reasonable fee. Since there is no ceiling on the total volume of services and there is only a limited fund created by the pooled capitation from which to make payment, beyond a certain point the dollar amount of payment for individual services must vary inversely with total utilization. Participating physicians therefore agree to prorate their fees when full payment would exhaust the capitation pool prematurely. The physicians are thus put at risk and are thereby motivated to be sparing in their use of services and facilities. They are assisted in this by the FMC's or HMO/IPA's ongoing review system.

The FMCs have much more to offer than economy, important though that may be. They inform their participating physicians of local health care issues and involve them in their solution. They involve physicians directly in the planning and improvement of program benefits. Finally, they make it possible for purchasers of service to negotiate with the physicians of a given area as a group, which cannot otherwise be done.

In summary, medical care foundations can bring to health care a management element, in the business sense, that is deficient or lacking in most current delivery systems. The HMO/IPA concept permits a number of combinations and permutations as far as participation by physician groups and carriers is concerned. A single HMO could contract with several IPAs and, conversely, a single IPA could contract with more than one HMO. The entire concept presented herein is not incompatible with Ellwood's recent proposals for the formation of health care alliances. Indeed, the building blocks of such alliances, as far as medical care and review are concerned, would have to be the FMCs, the IPAs, with or without HMOs, and the PSROs.

Peer review and the structuring of health care delivery along FMC and IPA lines are not proposed as panaceas for all the ills of our current system or systems, nor are they necessarily the only organizational types for review, data acquisition, planning, cost control, and delivery of services that might be explored. They do, however, have the capacity to support an orderly program of planning and implementation. Together, they constitute an organized, functioning, competent, and immediately available resource that can help to solve current problems and make substantial contributions to the ultimate development and operation of more rational health care delivery and financing systems.

Health professionals, industry, the carriers, and others of the private sector can no longer afford to sit by and meekly accept programs and administrative fiats from government since there is no reason to expect them to be less disastrous in the future than they have been in the past. There is an opportunity *now* to design and construct health care and payment systems that can be effective in a national program and to suggest them forcefully to government before the inevitable national health insurance legislation is cast in a monolith of concrete.

Contracting with an Independent Medical Organization for Corporate Health Programs

Stanley P. deLisser

11

Corporate health programs for employees and their families can have an important impact on reshaping the health delivery system by defining the issues and providing leadership for the nation's health planners. The real issues in health care are cost containment, increased access to primary care, realization that registered nurses are an underutilized resource, and recognition that our populace should seek an *optimal* health condition but not *unlimited* health care. Corporate programs to provide leadership will emphasize "primary care" which can be defined as embracing health education, preventive medicine, health maintenance, and counseling. (In this context, "corporate" is not limited to business corporations, but includes nonprofit organizations, union/management welfare funds, and government agencies at all levels.)

Many of us believe that the political controversies and actions of various interest groups have considerably muddled the real issues in health care and that clear understanding is lacking. I have several strong views that some may consider provocative: The first of these is that the best route to cost containment is increased competition. A major reason for skyrocketing costs is the lack of price sensitivity among doctors and hospitals. If individuals could exercise a choice among competing health providers for their health care dollar, the attitudes of doctors and hospitals would change markedly. This competition can be brought about by encouraging private industry to invest in the field and *make a profit.* We must do away with the obsolete notion that health care should be nonprofit. In fact, nonprofit organizations often deliver very expensive health care with no great emphasis on consumer satisfaction.

How do we get crisp, efficient management of health care facilities—skilled, cost-conscious management like General Motors or IBM, management concerned about customer service and satisfaction like MacDonalds or Holiday Inns? We get that kind of management by offering a profit motive, not by trying to exclude "profiteers" and keeping health care a private preserve for nonprofit institutions. One of our worst problems is the restrictive legislation and "keep out" atmosphere that limits the interest of profit-making organizations in offering competitive, innovative programs.

My second belief is that the availability of surgery and specialist care is really not a serious problem in the United States. Distribution is poor and planning agencies are attacking this problem. But our real lack is in primary care—someone to talk to about a problem, learning good health habits, somewhere to go with a sick child, a fever, a worrisome pain, screening of meaningful disease from the barrage of functional complaints, understanding of what good health really means and the personal responsibility for achieving it. In this area, corporate programs with their traditional emphasis on prevention and shift maintenance can be especially effective. However, I also believe that primary care can be rapidly expanded through a recognition that the principal provider of primary care should be the registered nurse, not the physician. Some experts believe that as much as 75 percent of all the care now rendered by family practitioners and internists could be effectively provided by registered nurses. Nurses could perform a lesser but still very significant proportion of the care now rendered by dermatologists, ophthalmologists, gynecologists, and several other specialties. The sheer waste of physician time dealing with the "worried well" is proportionately comparable to our country's profligate waste of energy. Nurses should be appropriately trained, supervised, and accorded the image and status with patients that is necessary. Consider the potential savings in doctor time! Consider the fact that there are estimated to be over 350,000 trained RNs who are not actively practicing owing to family commitments or other inability to work full time! Consider that over 50 percent of these nurses would like to work on a part-time basis! We should stop experimenting with physicians' associates, Medex, and so on, and realize that our single greatest resource for broadening primary care *with almost no investment* is the registered nurse.

Finally, I believe that we must deemphasize the role of hospitals as the principal institution in reshaping our health delivery system. We need a vast new expansion of ambulatory care units concentrating on primary care. Hospitals are unwieldy bureaucracies, torn by conflicting interests, dominated by patient care decisions of physicians that are often self-serving, overlorded by lay boards which are usually more social than effective. How can such institutions be expected to extend out into the community and establish small, RN-staffed, ambulatory primary care units? But corporations can! For their own employees and families as well as for a business offering services on a competitive basis.

A cost-effective primary care extended plan for employees can be implemented through an in-house department or an independent medical service contractor. There are a handful of companies that have been doing this for many years—Consolidated Edison in New York comes immediately to mind. Of late, there seems to be an increasing number of corporations that are extending programs or at least talking about it. To the best of my knowledge, most of the interest has occurred where there is an aggressive, forward-looking medical director who pushes management. Gil Collings at New York Telephone and Allen Garb at Squibb are acquaintances of mine in New York who seem to provide this kind of leadership. More often than not, this type of medical director is not a "health planner" who is overly concerned about the national scene. Usually, he is a clinician who is turned off by the indifferent quality of care that he sees being received by employees who come to him for counsel.

Those of us who have worked for many years in direct patient care in the occupational setting have an excellent window through which to see the quality of care rendered by the private medical sector. To put it mildly indeed, the quality of care is often less than inspiring. The sacred institutions of "family doctor," "free choice of physician," and "our community hospital" frequently do not perform at anywhere near the level perceived by patients. Patient perception is vitally important. If the employee believes that his family doctor is God and the plant physician is "a jerk who couldn't make a living in private practice," how valuable can the extended corporate program ever be? Unstinting insistence on quality care and patient-doctor communication (the "art of medicine") is a cornerstone that must be in place. Here again, the nurse is often more effective than the physician. I am amazed at the awe in which patients view their doctors. They are in the presence of the Great Man and very often their anxiety precludes any real understanding of what the doctor said, much less the nurse.

Can a corporate program be extended to cover the full range of medical and hospital services? It is very difficult. The normal scatter pattern of employee residences, the frequency of long-distance commuting, restrictive legislation, and other factors work against an all-inclusive plan. A more promising approach is simply an extension of the primary care aspects of the occupational health programs. Although everyone in occupational health is now very OSHA-sensitive, any worthwhile program has contained for many years a number of aspects of primary care: personal health counseling, health education, "sick call" facilities for early diagnosis and minor treatment, and a wide range of preventive medicine activities from immunizations to comprehensive periodic physical examinations. The more advanced programs are acutely aware of the destructive effects of stress overload and offer various psychiatric and counseling services. In particular, services to combat alcoholism and drug abuse are in effect.

However, these primary care programs are seldom offered to dependents, principally because of cost. Corporate management has been very slow to "invest" in extended programs owing to a lack of conviction that the investment will pay off and not just be another addition to overhead expense. This is quite understandable—there has been little or no solid evidence to support the case for the investment. Also, there has been a strange reluctance to get involved with the general medical care system. "We have insurance for that," says the executive. It should be clear by now that if the cost of health care skyrockets, the cost of the corporation's health insurance will skyrocket as well. The bridge between the occupational health program and the employee benefit program must be crossed. There is a very definite relationship between them. The opportunity for extending the occupational health program to provide some of the services covered under the employee benefit program is worth considering—particularly because both improved quality and cost containment results are possible.

Specifically, I am proposing that corporations extend their occupational health programs, either through an in-house medical department or an outside health services contractor as follows:

Policy definition that there is a corporate role in primary care for employees and dependents.

Refinement and improvement of primary care services offered to employees. In particular, there must be a strong health counseling service available.

Extension of primary care services to dependents, recognizing that logistical factors may have a limiting effect.

Providing for seven-day a week, 24-hour a day access to small units staffed by one or two nurses. These units should be located near employee residence concentrations.

When operating their own primary care nursing units is impractical, corporations should band together to operate such units.

If corporations prefer to use independent contractors to operate these primary care units, there are plenty of able clinics and physician entrepreneurs available. If not, call us; we will do it for you.

Through their employee benefit plans and corporate medical departments, corporations are ideally positioned to bring about these changes. Employees will utilize whatever type of health care system employers provide, either directly or by the terms of their health insurance plans. If a corporate Blue Cross plan will not pay for diagnostic x-rays except for hospital inpatients, employees and their families will go into the hospital to get them. If the plan provides outpatient care, they will not go into the hospital. If the in-house medical department offers periodic checkups, employees will come and participate. However, a much smaller percentage will do so if they have to seek out their family doctor and write out a check for the service. A highly effective method of health education is to provide the American worker with a health benefit he does not have to pay for in cash.

The object of aggressively offering primary care is to provide employees and dependents with a quality-controlled alternative to the existing system. The mere fact of such programs' coming into being will put pressure on private physicians and hospitals to operate more effectively and think twice about pricing. However, only a small percentage of corporate groups can offer reasonably comprehensive in-house health care. Most will want to turn to outside providers: local physicians, HMOs, hospitals, or independent medical organizations such as EHE Health Services, Inc.

Cost Containment through Benefit Plan Design

Henry A. DiPrite

12

The cost of health care is far outpacing the general rate of inflation and already has reached unacceptable levels. The $69 billion spent for health care in 1970 increased to almost twice that amount in 1976 and is projected by the Department of Health, Education, and Welfare to exceed $240 billion by 1982. Health care expenditures in 1976 represented 8.6 percent of gross national product. This was up from 5.9 percent in 1967 and, left unchecked, will exceed 10 percent by 1982. These unhealthy rates of health care cost inflation translate into ever-increased health insurance premiums to employer and employee alike, and to higher taxes and consumer out-of-pocket payments. Inexorably, year after year, each citizen is being forced to allocate more and more of his or her income for questionable added health care value.

The purpose of this paper is briefly to review some of the principal factors contributing to rising health care costs and some current cost-control strategies, particularly those which are closely related to the third-party financing system; and then to explore in detail a series of benefit modifications that can be used to reduce both premium rates and claims costs.

Third-Party Influence in Benefit Plan Design

To comprehend the problems associated with rising health care costs, and hence the more plausible ways of dampening their rise, requires an understanding of the health care system's complexity. To illustrate:

> Ninety percent of hospital services are paid for by a third party such as the federal government, state governments, private insurers, or Blue Cross. Under this system, neither the patient nor the provider feels any noticeable economic pressure at the time the service is delivered.[1]

> The present system of hospital cost reimbursement repays hospitals for the costs they have incurred. This automatic pass-through system does not contain proper incentives for efficient management.

> Both patients and providers expect unlimited resources to be available for treatment of an illness no matter how great the costs. Advancing medical technology can offer esoteric incremental benefits of sometimes marginal value at outlandish costs. So long as someone else pays for it, every patient wants the newest "add-on."

> Malpractice liability is of growing financial concern, in part because of increased patient expectations. It results in a twofold problem: a significant increase in malpractice insurance premiums charged providers of service which much be passed through to payers; and, even more importantly, major increases in defensive medical practice to minimize the possibility of lawsuits. Some students of the current scene estimate as much as 5 percent of total medical care costs are solely for defensive medical purposes.[2]

> Under the various mixed public-private health care cost reimbursement systems in effect in this country, what cost controls there are have limited impact on cost containment. Reduction in reimbursements by Medicare only shifts costs to other payers. Disallowance of certain costs by one private sector source of payment shifts reimbursements for costs already expended to other sources of payment.

To be effective, cost containment solutions, whether now operative or proposed, must recognize these causal factors and work to minimize or remove them.

Improving Benefit Plan Design and Implementation

The rationale for the cost containment ideas that follow lies in a hypothesis born over the years of cost containment experience, failure, change, and then partial success. This hypothesis contends that any significant success in reducing the rate of health care inflation must combine legislative action to cover areas where voluntary actions are illegal, impractical, or ineffective, with vigorous private sector action through individual efforts of the major insurers and providers.

It is an unfortunate fact of life that major effective containment of health care costs cannot be achieved without fundamental new legislation and rule-making at both the state and federal levels. Major needs include prompt implementation of the 1976 Health Maintenance Organization Amendments to improve the chances for success of this viable alternative form of health care delivery. Also needed is nationwide passage of prospective institutional budget review legislation. A system such as that installed in Connecticut and Maryland can save substantial money through rate review and budget approval without unreasonable impact on hospitals. Under prospective budget review, hospitals are required to budget in the same way as other businesses and set charges accordingly.

Legislation should also extend professional standards review organizations (PSROs) and other peer review mechanisms that monitor hospital and physician services for patients under governmental programs to cover such services for all patients, regardless of type of payer—public or private. Already there is mounting evidence that by controlling quality, the PSRO mechanism works to contain costs.[3] An additional provision of such legislation could be authorization to set PSRO standards by patient condition for appropriate tests and procedures. Such criteria could be most useful for defense in medical malpractice suits.

Legislation is also needed for hospitals, requiring them to accept tests done by qualified outside laboratories to eliminate redundant and expensive retesting, and to charge in-house test rates that are reasonable in relation to the rates of qualified independent laboratories in the community. It should prohibit third-party payer reinbursement for use of any facilities obtainable without certificate of need. If accredited health planning agency decisions determine a facility or service is not necessary, then providers should not be reimbursed for that service.

Legislation standardizing and expanding paramedical licensing laws would encourage this necessary, less costly form of physician-supervised medical care. Legislation should also limit by geographic area the kinds and amounts of medical equipment, including out-of-hospital equipment. Expensive CAT scanners are one example of potentially overused and expensive equipment. Geographic limits on the number of residents in the various specialties would serve to increase the availability of family doctors to underserved communities.

Limited enabling legislation should be passed to allow experimentation with collecting and publishing provider charge data by geographic area for representative medical and dental procedures. Broad availability of such data would encourage consumers to become more aware of medical fees generally and, ideally, to discuss fees in advance with their physicians and dentists. Enabling legislation should also allow collective negotiation with physicians for reasonable and customary fee arrangements whereby the provider agrees to accept the reimbursement as payment in full. Such an arrangement would assure that patients will not have to bear charges above what insurers reimburse as reasonable and customary.

Even with extensive health care cost containment legislation, voluntary private sector action is essential for the overall system to work effectively. To this end, considerable progress already has been achieved. Some recent developments include preadmission testing—a concept whereby insurance reimburses a patient for necessary preliminary testing on an outpatient basis before hospitalization, thus reducing the expensive inpatient confinement expense. This concept should work even better as more doctors become aware of its existence and encourage their patients to use it. Another trend is in programs for a second opinion before surgery. A growing number of group plans provide for reimbursement of costs for a second or even third medical opinion for elective surgery. Evidence suggests a real potential for significant hospital and surgical cost savings by reducing the rate of unnecessary operations.[4]

The less expensive outpatient form of care is being encouraged by including health insurance reimbursement for ambulatory surgical care for minor surgery, which can be safe and far less expensive than inpatient surgery, and skilled nursing facility care and home health care for necessary recuperation on a less expensive basis than in-hospital. Other favorable developments in insurance include reasonable coinsurance and deductible features to motivate the patient to avoid overuse of health care facilities and services, and reimbursement for properly supervised paramedical services to improve physicians' productivity and lower costs without impairing quality. The challenge here is to educate the patient to accept the paramedic as a physician-substitute in the provision of routine treatment.

There is also a growing emphasis on the importance of preventive maintenance. An excellent example is the rapid expansion of group dental insurance including prophylaxis and examination. Less well known is the beginning of coverage for periodic physical examinations. Another insurance development is the coordination of benefits (COB) provision under group health insurance plans. This industry-wide provision eliminates overpayment of medical bills when a patient is insured under more than one health care plan. John Hancock estimates that in 1976 it passed on to group policyholders COB savings of over $10 million.

Despite the progress already made, the private sector can and must do more. We in the group insurance industry are experimenting with further ways to contain costs while continuing sound coverage to employees and their dependents. A possible approach lies in encouraging employers to redesign their health care insurance plans. Despite obvious administrative and labor-management bargaining limitations, I believe that somewhere in these United States there exist employers with all the right conditions to be daring enough, with the help of group insurers, to experiment with alternative benefit plan designs in order to effect cost-saving modifications. Here are some illustrations of what I mean.

Benefit Modifications That Result in Reduction of Premium Rates

The employer's cost for a particular plan can be reduced by making the employee responsible for budgetable deductible and coinsurance amounts in exchange for protection against a catastrophic financial loss from severe injury or sickness. This shifting of emphasis from first-dollar benefits to protection against catastrophic loss assumes that the family budget should provide for routine medical expenses. The wage earner might be more prudent in procuring his or her family's health care services where first-dollar expenses must be paid out of pocket. The result is a reduction in claim costs and premium rates.

A typical plan of group health insurance consists of a full-service plan of basic hospital and medical benefits supplemented by major medical insurance with a $100 per calendar year deductible and a $50,000 lifetime maximum. Under this plan, the employee is not responsible for the first-dollar base plan expenses and thus has no monetary incentive for utilizing less costly alternative forms of health care. The only incentives for cost savings are the minimal major medical deductible and coinsurance.

The following exhibits illustrate the approximate reduction in the premium rate, rounded to the nearest half-percent, of a typical plan that results from certain benefit plan modifications. (The composite premium rate used as the basis for reduction assumes a 75 percent dependent enrollment and the nationwide average for reasonable and customary surgical fees and semiprivate hospital room charges.) The exhibits also indicate the approximate percentage increase in the premium rate resulting from the addition of major medical catastrophic options. Presently, the standard catastrophic options limit an individual's annual out-of-pocket expenses because of the application of the major medical deductible and coinsurance to $500 or $1,000. A family annual out-of-pocket maximum is presented in the exhibits, to show the relatively large approximate percentage increase in the plan's premium required by this type of modification. The actual amount of premium reduction for each of these benefit modifications will depend on individual case characteristics. Thus, the exhibits are for demonstration purposes only, and the illustrated reductions are only approximations.

Exhibit 1 suggests how a rich base plan supplemented by major medical can be modified to make the employee more financially responsible for the family's health care expenses. The suggested plan changes and resulting approximate reduction in the premium rate are displayed for each kind of coverage. An estimate of the overall premium reduction can be derived by merely adding the percentage reductions displayed for each benefit modification selected. If the catastrophic major medical option is added, the overall estimated premium rate reduction will be decreased by the additional premium cost displayed for this option.

Before implementing benefit modifications of the kinds illustrated, some practical procedures should be considered. For instance, a decision to set the benefit maximum at 70 percent or 80 percent of reasonable and customary charges would require additional manual computation under a computer-oriented claim-processing system and may result in additional administrative costs. A second consideration is employee cost-sharing. One alternative displayed for base plan modifications lists the percentage of premium reduction expected if expenses exceeding the modified limit are not considered a covered major medical expense. For example, charges in excess of 80 percent of reasonable and customary, or hospital charges in excess of the $5,000 unallocated maximum would not be covered under the supplemental major medical and, therefore, would be the responsibility of the employee. This approach is not recommended as a practical alternative since an extreme financial hardship could be imposed on the employee in the event of severe illness or injury.

Calendar year major medical plans contain a standard "carry-over" provision to the effect that covered expenses incurred in the last three months of a calendar year used to satisfy the deductible for that year will be carried forward to satisfy the next calendar year's deductible. If the deductible accumulation period is reduced to less than three months, a conflict between the three-month carry-over provision and the accumulation period will arise. For example, assume the deductible accumulation period for a calendar year plan (with the standard three-month carry-over) is reduced to one month. Prior to this change, a charge incurred on November 15 and used to satisfy the deductible in the year incurred would be eligible to be carried over into the next year to satisfy that year's deductible. Since the accumulation period commences on November 15, the deductible amount would have to be satisfied by December 15, because of the one-month accumulation period, and would not be carried over. This change may cause concern among the employees. A suggested solution is to limit the carry-over period to the lesser of three months or the length of the deductible accumulation period.

Exhibit 2 displays approximate premium reductions that can be realized by modifying an in-force comprehensive major medical plan. It should be noted that, unlike in exhibit 1, the effect on the overall premium rate reduction from selecting more than one modification will generally be greater than that from adding the corresponding premium rate reductions for each modification selected. This is caused by the interaction of the two modifications on the coverage. If the plan under consideration is identical to the one described in exhibit 2, except that the deductible amount is $50, the percentage reduction in the premium rate obtained by increasing the deductible to $100 is 11 percent. The effect of any further modifications can then be added to this percentage to estimate the overall reduction.

Exhibit 3 demonstrates approximate reductions in premium rate resulting from both increasing the deductible amount and reducing the accumulation period of the plan described in exhibit 2. This percentage can be added to any coinsurance modifications displayed in exhibit 2 to arrive at an approximation of the overall premium rate reduction for a comprehensive-type plan.

Ways of modifying the two traditional approaches of providing health insurance, namely, a base plan supplemented by major medical and comprehensive major medical, have been presented in exhibits 1, 2, and 3. By adding a

Exhibit 1
Approximate Reductions in Premium Rates Resulting from Modification of Benefit Provisions

In-force plan

Description of benefits

Hospital expense benefits

Room: Semiprivate
Duration: 120 Days
Special services: Unlimited

Benefit Modification	Approximate Percent Reduction in Composite Premium Rate
I. Add Front-End Deductible Applicable to Hospital Charges, per period of disability. Not a Covered Major Medical Expense.	
$ 25	1.5%
$ 50	2.5%
$100	3.5%
$150	4.0%
$200	5.0%
II. Change to Unallocated Hospital Maximum of $5,000 Semiprivate Room; Excess Charges, if any:	
Covered Major Medical Expense	1.0%
Not Covered Major Medical Expense	4.5%
III. Change to Fixed Dollar-Room Limit of Approximately 80% of Semiprivate or 80% of the actual Semiprivate Room Charge; 120 days duration; Special Services— 80% of reasonable and customary; Excess Charges, if any;	
Covered Major Medical Expense	2.5%
Not Covered Major Medical Expense	7.5%
IV. Same as Modification III, only change Special Hospital Services to 100% of the First $2,000 of reasonable and customary charges; Excess Charges, if any:	
Covered Major Medical Expense	2.5%
Not Covered Major Medical Expense	8.5%

[Continued]

Exhibit 1 [*Continued*]
Approximate Reductions in Premium Rates Resulting from Modification of Benefit Provisions

In-force plan

Description of benefits

Surgical expense benefits
Reasonable & customary

Medical expense benefits
In-hospital $8/day for 120 days

Diagnostic x-ray and laboratory expense benefits
$100 calendar year maximum

	Benefit Modification	*Approximate Percent Reduction in Composite Premium Rate*
V.	Change Surgical to Scheduled Amount approximately 80% of reasonable and customary or 80% of the actual reasonable and customary charge; Excess Charges, if any:	
	Covered Major Medical Expense	1.0%
	Not Covered Major Medical Expense	3.0%
VI.	Change Surgical to Scheduled Amount approximately 70% of reasonable and customary or 70% of the actual reasonable and customary charge; Excess Charges, if any:	
	Covered Major Medical Expense	2.0%
	Not Covered Major Medical Expense	4.5%
VII.	Medical Charges covered only as Major Medical Expense	1.0%
VIII.	X-Ray and Laboratory charges covered only as Major Medical Expenses	1.0%

front-end deductible and introducing elements of coinsurance through setting the maximum benefit at 80 percent of reasonable and customary, the base plus supplemental approach begins to resemble the comprehensive concept.

The comprehensive concept is probably easier to explain to employees and to administer. For example, it may be difficult to explain to an employee insured under a base plus supplemental major medical plan that, after a front-end deductible for each period of disability, he or she will be reimbursed 80 percent of reasonable and customary charges incurred under the base plan. The insured individual then must accumulate within one month the amount necessary to satisfy a calendar year major medical deductible. After doing so, the

Exhibit 1 [*Continued*]
Approximate Reductions in Premium Rates Resulting from Modification of Benefit Provisions

In-force plan
Description of benefits
Supplemental major medical expense benefits
Calendar year plan

Deductible: $100 applied to a maximum of 2 family members
Accumulation period: 12 months
3 month carry-over provision

Coinsurance: 80%/20%
Mental illness: 50%/50%
$10 Visit; $500/calendar year

Maximum: $50,000 lifetime with reinstatement

Benefit Modification	Approximate Percent Reduction in Composite Premium Rate
IX. Reduce Accumulation Period to	
6 Months	3.0%
3 Months	4.5%
1 Month	9.0%

Benefit Modification	Approximate Percent Increase in Composite Premium Rate
X. Add Catastrophic Option; Maximum out-of-pocket expenses from application of Major Medical Deductible and coinsurance amounts:	
$1,000/Individual	3.5%
$ 500/Individual	4.0%
$1,000/Family	7.0%

individual will be reimbursed 80 percent of the remaining 20 percent of reasonable and customary charges not payable under the base plan. The employee's maximum out-of-pocket expenses in any calendar year owing to the application of the major medical deductible and coinsurance might be as much as $500.

Thus, exhibit 4 describes the essentials of various comprehensive-type plans arranged according to the approximate percentage of premium saved compared with the in-force premium for the plan defined in exhibit 2. Alternative experiments could be conducted with varying amounts of coinsurance subject to a proper catastrophic payout limit for the covered individual. Insur-

Exhibit 2
Approximate Reductions in Premium Rates Resulting from Modification of Benefit Provisions

In-force plan
Description of benefits
Comprehensive major medical expense benefits
Calendar Year Plan

Deductible: $100 per individual, applied to a maximum of 2 family members, waived on hospital and surgical charges
Accumulation period: 12 months 3 month carry-over provision

Coinsurance: 80%/20%, waived on the first $5,000 of hospital charges
Mental illness: 50%/50%; $10/visit; $500/calendar year

Maximum: $50,000 lifetime with reinstatement

Benefit Modification	Approximate Percent Reduction In Composite Premium Rate	
I. Waive $100 deductible for hospital charges only	6.0%	
II. No waivers of $100 deductible	14.5%	
III. Reduce Accumulation Period of $100 deductible to:		
6 Months	3.0%	
3 Months	5.5%	
1 Month	11.0%	
	Waived on Hosp and Surg	*No Waivers*
IV. Increase Deductible Amount to:		
$150 per individual	2.0%	20.0%
$200 per individual	4.0%	26.5%
$250 per individual	5.0%	30.5%
$500 per individual	8.0%	50.0%
$500 per family	2.5%	23.0%
$1,000 per family	5.5%	37.0%
$250 per individual with a $500 maximum for all family members	2.5%	21.0%

Benefit Modification	Approximate Percent Reduction in Composite Premium Rate
V. Waive Coinsurance on Hospital Charges Only for the following amounts:	
$2,000	1.0%
$1,000	2.5%
$ 500	4.5%
VI. No Waivers of Coinsurance	8.0%

Exhibit 2 [Continued]
Approximate Reductions in Premium Rates Resulting from Modification of Benefit Provisions

VII. Add Catastrophic Option Maximum out-of-pocket expenses from application of Major Medical Deductible and Coinsurance amounts:	Approximate Percent Increase In Composite Premium Rate
$1,000/Individual	4.0%
$ 500/Individual	4.5%
$1,000/Family	7.5%

ers must stand ready to respond to interested employers with systems and underwriting innovations as well as flexible administrative practices.

Some additional cost containment measures which require further analysis to determine their practical application and the degree of claim savings, if any, can be suggested. One of these would be to transfer the benefit for the administration of anesthesia from hospital special services to surgical coverage and limit the maximum anesthesia benefit to a percentage of the scheduled surgical maximum. Traditionally, this limit has been 20 percent of the scheduled surgical maximum, but recent evidence indicates that anesthesia charges are increasing in relation to surgical charges. A limit of 40 percent to 50 percent might be a more practical consideration. This modification could introduce a greater degree of employee cost-sharing for anesthesia expenses.

A second cost containment measure would permit the insured to enter directly into an extended care facility as an alternative to hospital confinement. This direct admission for nonsurgical care would have to be certified as medically necessary by the attending physician and be recertified every seven days. Another alternative to inpatient care would permit the insured individual

Exhibit 3
Approximate Reductions in Premium Rates Resulting from Increasing the $100 Deductible and Reducing the 12 Month Accumulation Period of the Comprehensive Major Medical Plan in Exhibit 2

Accumulation Period	Deductible Amount—Waived on Hospital and Surgical Charges			
	$100	$150	$200	$250
12 Months	—	2.0%	4.0%	5.0%
6 Months	3.0%	4.5%	7.5%	8.5%
3 Months	5.5%	8.0%	11.0%	12.0%
1 Month	11.0%	13.5%	16.5%	17.0%

Exhibit 4
Description of Plan Essentials That Effect a Premium Savings of Approximately 5% of the In-Force Premium for the Plan Defined in Exhibit 2

	Deductible	Coinsurance	Maximum	Approx. Savings
I.	$100 Waived on Hospital 2 family members 12-month accum. period	80%/20% Waived on First $500 of Hospital Mental Illness 50%/50%	Unlimited Cat. Option $500/ Individual	5.5%
II.	$150 Waived on Hosp & Surg 2 family members 12-month accum. period	80%/20% Waived on First $500 of Hospital Mental Illness 50%/50%	$50,000 Lifetime	6.0%
III.	$100 Waived on Hosp & Surg 2 family members 1-month accum. period	80%/20% Waived on First $5,000 of Hospital Mental Illness 50%/50%	Unlimited Cat. Option $500/ Individual	6.5%
IV.	$200 Waived on Hosp & Surg 2 family members 3-month accum. period	80%/20% Waived on First $5,000 of Hospital Mental Illness 50%/50%	Unlimited Cat. Option $500/ Individual	6.5%
V.	$150 Waived on Hosp & Surg 2 family members 3-month accum. period	80%/20% Waived on First $1,000 of Hospital Mental Illness 50%/50%	Unlimited Cat. Option $500/ Individual	6.0%

Description of Plan Essentials That Effect a Premium Savings of Approximately 10% of the In-Force Premium for the Plan Defined in Exhibit 2

I.	$100 No Waivers 2 family members 12-month accum. period	80%/20% Waived on First $5,000 of Hospital Mental Illness 50%/50%	Unlimited Cat. Option $500/Individual	10.0%
II.	$100 Waived on Hospital 2 family members 12-month accum. period	80%/20% Waived on First $500 of Hospital Mental Illness 50%/50%	$50,000 Lifetime	10.0%
III.	$100 Waived on Hosp & Surg 2 family members 6-month accum. period	80%/20% Mental Illness 50%/50%	$50,000 Lifetime	10.5%
IV.	$100 Waived on Hospital 2 family members 6-month accum. period	80%/20% Waived on First $1,000 of Hospital Mental Illness 50%/50%	$50,000 Lifetime	10.0%

Description of Plan Essentials That Effect a Premium Savings of Approximately *15%* of the In-Force Premium for the Plan Defined in Exhibit 2

I.	$100 Waived on Hospital 2 family members 6-month accum. period	80%/20% Mental Illness 50%/50%	$50,000 Lifetime	16.0%
II.	$200 Waived on Hosp & Surg 2 family members 3-month accum. period	80%/20% Waived on First $500 of Hospital Mental Illness 50%/50%	$50,000 Lifetime	15.5%
III.	$200 Waived on Hosp & Surg 2 family members 3-month accum. period	80%/20% Mental Illness 50%/50%	Unlimited Cat. Option $1,000/Individual	15.0%
IV.	$100 Waived on Hospital 2 family members 1-month accum. period	80%/20% Waived on First $1,000 of Hospital Mental Illness 50%/50%	Unlimited Cat. Option $500/Individual	14.0%

[Continued]

Exhibit 4 [Continued]
Description of Plan Essentials That Effect a Premium Savings of Approximately 5% of the In-Force Premium for the Plan Defined in Exhibit 2

	Deductible	Coinsurance	Maximum	Approx. Savings
V.	$150 No Waivers 2 family members 12-month accum. period	80%/20% Waived on First $5,000 of Hospital Mental Illness 50%/50%	Unlimited Cat. Option $500/ Individual	15.5%

Description of Plan Essentials That Effect a Premium Savings of Approximately 20% of the In-Force Premium for the Plan Defined in Exhibit 2

	Deductible	Coinsurance	Maximum	Approx. Savings
I.	$100 No Waivers 2 family members 6-month accum. period	80%/20% Mental Illness 50%/50%	Unlimited Cat. Option $500/ Individual	20.0%
II.	$150 No Waivers 2 family members 12-month accum. period	80%/20% Mental Illness 50%/50%	Unlimited Cat. Option $1,000/ Family	20.0%
III.	$100 Waived on Hospital 2 family members 1-month accum. period	80%/20% Waived on First $500 of Hospital Mental Illness 50%/50%	$50,000 Lifetime	20.5%
IV.	$100 Waived on Hospital 2 family members 1-month accum. period	80%/20% Mental Illness 50%/50%	Unlimited Cat. Option $500/ Individual	19.0%
V.	$200 No Waivers	80%/20% Waived on First	Unlimited Cat.	19.0%

| | 2 family members 12-month accum. period | $5,000 of Hospital Mental Illness 50%/50% | Option $1,000/ Family | |

Description of Plan Essentials That Effect a Premium Savings of Approximately 30% of the In-Force Premium for the Plan Defined in Exhibit 2

I.	$200 No Waivers 2 family members 12-month accum. period	80%/20% Mental Illness 50%/50%	Unlimited Cat. Option $1,000/ Individual	30.5%
II.	$250 No Waivers 2 family members 12-month accum. period	80%/20% Waived on First $500 of Hospital Mental Illness 50%/50%	Unlimited Cat. Option $500/ Individual	30.0%
III.	$200 No Waivers 2 family members 6-month accum. period	80%/20% Waived on First $5,000 of Hospital Mental Illness 50%/50%	Unlimited Cat. Option $1,000/ Family	29.5%
IV.	$500 Cumulative No Waivers 12-month accum. period	80%/20% Mental Illness 50%/50%	$50,000 Lifetime	31.0%
V.	$250 Individual $500 Cumulative No Waivers 12-month accum. period	80%/20% Mental Illness 50%/50%	$50,000 Lifetime	28.5%

Description of Plan Essentials That Effect a Premium Savings of Approximately 40% of the In-Force Premium for the Plan Defined in Exhibit 2

I.	$250 No Waivers 2 family members 6-month accum. period	80%/20% Mental Illness 50%/50%	$50,000 Lifetime	40.5%

[Continued]

Exhibit 4 [Continued]
Description of Plan Essentials That Effect a Premium Savings of Approximately 5% of the In-Force Premium for the Plan Defined in Exhibit 2

	Deductible	Coinsurance	Maximum	Approx. Savings
II.	$250 No Waivers 2 family members 3-month accum. period	80%/20% Mental Illness 50%/50%	Unlimited Cat. Option $500/ Individual	38.5%
III.	$1,000 Family No Waivers 12-month accum. period	80%/20% Mental Illness 50%/50%	Unlimited Cat. Option $1,000/ Family	37.0%

Description of Plan Essentials That Effect a Premium Savings of Approximately 50% of the In-Force Premium for the Plan Defined in Exhibit 2

	Deductible	Coinsurance	Maximum	Approx. Savings
I.	$500 No Waivers 2 family members 12-month accum. period	80%/20% Mental Illness 50%/50%	Unlimited Cat. Option $1,000/ Family	50.0%

to utilize ambulatory surgical facilities or extended care facilities in lieu of more costly inpatient hospital care and pay the actual reasonable and customary charge with no deductible or coinsurance. This would encourage the patient to seek out less costly alternatives to hospital care.

Further, one could offer employees with different financial and family circumstances a choice of alternative deductible amounts. For example, the deductible could be related to income. In addition to the expected premium and claim savings, employees and dependents with their deductibles "on the line" may exert a cost-containing influence where a third party payer could not. In order for such an innovation to be credible, the employees must be assured that any premium and claim savings will be used to their direct benefit in the form of an additional benefit or a wage supplement.

Finally, efforts should be accelerated in consumer and provider education as to why various cost containment devices in the long run serve the self-interest of each of us, with actual examples of cost savings. Equally important are combined provider, insurer, and governmental campaigns of "good health" education directed to the general public. It must be made clear that incremental dollars for new esoteric medical benefits will do less to improve the level of health than a proper diet, sufficient exercise, avoidance of smoking and excess alcohol, and other sensible practices requiring individual responsibility. Without such self-restraint, "good health" will continue to elude our citizenry no matter what amount we spend on health care.

These cost containment measures might be handled on an experimental basis with the cooperation of the medical profession and insurers in selected areas allowing for close monitoring of results. Of course, a proper appeal mechanism through recognized peer review would have to exist. It seems far better to gain experience in the area of cost control by voluntarily experimenting within the private sector on a limited basis than by plunging into a mandated, untested, across-the-board national solution.

NOTES

1. M. Mueller and R. Gibson, "National Health Expenditures, Fiscal Year 1975," *Social Security Bulletin*, February 1976, pp. 3–20.

2. "The Skyrocketing Cost of Health Care," *Business Week*, May 17, 1976, pp. 144–148.

3. "Report of PSRO Performance: A Limited Survey," Health Insurance Association of America, 1975.

4. Eugene McCarthy, M.D., and Ann Susan Kamons, "Voluntary and Mandatory Presurgical Screening Programs: An Analysis of their Implications," presented to the American Federation for Clinical Research, May 2, 1976; and Norman Miller, M.D., "Hysterectomy: Therapeutic Necessity or Surgical Racket," *American Journal of Obstetrics and Gynecology* 51:804–810, June 1976.

Monitoring the Quality of Health Care Services

Henry C. Damm and Karl Bunkelman

13

The cost of health services has been increasing exponentially over the last decade, with an unknown effect on the quality of service rendered.[1] Despite the emergence of a variety of cost containment efforts by the ultimate purchasers of health services in industry, labor, and government, the ability to ascertain quality has eluded us. We are told, for example, of the decrease in utilization of surgery and lengths of stay resulting from experience with HMOs, second opinion programs, and PSRO-type activities, but a minimum of data exist to demonstrate any positive impact from these efforts on the health of the recipients of services.[2] Many industrial purchasers have had to increase the capabilities of in-house clinics because employees' nonoccupational health problems have not been adequately diagnosed or treated by outside providers. It is unknown exactly how many unnecessary dollars are being expended by in-house clinics in duplicating services already purchased through benefit plans.[3]

The purchasers of health services must have valid, continuous data in order to evaluate the services received. Only then can they know whether they are getting the best value for the dollar. They must be able to measure the effectiveness of any cost control approach and to know in advance what its trade-offs will be with quality. Outcomes of service can be measured statistically and actuarilly by their "spillover" effect on sick pay, disability benefits, Workmen's Compensation, death benefits, absenteeism, cost of retraining, and cost of rehabilitation.[4] Traditionally, purchasers in industry, labor, and government have not considered the total drain of their health dollar, that is, both medical and spillover costs. It would be most interesting to eventually be able to calculate the total impact of this drain on the gross national product, since it is not unrealistic to assume that upwards of $50 billion is being expended annually as a result of unnecessary and preventable costs and damage.

Although such factors as increased costs of technology, equipment, and personnel have contributed to the inflation of health costs, they do not begin to approach the massive increases owing to standards, not being followed by providers and to the lack of procedures to minimize errors. Damm and Associates' review of adverse medical service outcomes over the last seven years and the results of national studies including the Ribicoff Commission, the HEW Secretary's Commission on Malpractice, the American College of Surgeons' report on preventable incidents, and the National Association of Insurance Commissioners reports on malpractice indicate that somewhere between 20 and 40 percent of every health services dollar goes for unnecessary and preventable costs and/or damage.[5] It has been suggested that the individual employee should be the focus of cost control through copayment and deductibles. However, only 18 percent of health costs go for physicians' fees, with over 40 percent covering hospitals costs. Of preventable damage, 85 to 90 percent occurs in the hospital. There are some 7,000 hospitals and some 280,000 physicians. Therefore, from a cost-benefit standpoint it is obvious that the focus for cost and quality control should initially be on the hospital.[6]

Within the hospital cost spectrum are two areas that are draining purchasers' budgets unmercifully and yet there is very little known about their nature or the extent of their impact. The first is preventable damage, such as mental retardation, that is very high in per incident cost and, owing to public settlements and court awards, fairly well known, but is relatively low in frequency. Ineffective loss control programs by hospitals and their liability carriers perpetuate this kind of damage.[7] A much greater expense to the purchaser is preventable damage that is low in per incident cost but massive in frequency. An example is the hysterectomy that, through negligence, leads to infection and goes from a normal seven-day stay to one of thirty days. Such occurences and subsequent repair actions are usually not recorded on hospital incident report forms because of fear of reprisal or ignorance by the hospital staff. No liability claim is made, and these unnecessary costs are automatically included in the hospital bill to be paid again through higher insurance premiums the following year. It is estimated that no more than 15 to 25 percent of these compensable incidents are ever reported to permit future corrective action. Loss control programs have been either too superficial or too supplier-oriented to be of any value to the purchaser.[8]

Nebulous terms like "clinical judgment" and "quality of care" have been too often accepted as blanket justification for preventable and unnecessary costs and/or damages, despite the fact that health services can be measured in terms as precise as the industrial products being scrutinized every day through quality control systems. The concept is by no means new. Medical-legal measurement has historically been practiced by the American College of Legal Medicine under the common term *forensic medicine*. Forensic refers to the presenting of data for examination in a public forum, such as the courts. Over the years, medical literature and court decisions across the country have reverified medical center findings and have led to the emergence of national contract standards.[9] The standards that purchasers should be demanding are those that the providers indicate that they are already following. They purport to be adhering to the standards, rules, and regulations of some 800 boards and bodies, including the American Medical Association, the American College of Surgeons, and the American Hospital Association.[10] However, with the absence of a uniform measurement system using valid standard criteria, the purchasers' best cost reduction approach might well be to eliminate benefits altogether. Without standard criteria, any corporation would be totally unable to provide a uniform product to its customers and compete in a national market. This is a reasonable parallel with the state of provision of health services today.

The inconsistency in quality of health services being supplied to national purchasers, including Medicare and Medicaid, has resulted in a wide range of returns on investment, depending on the location of delivery. Developments such as PSROs have only exacerbated the situation; local review systems are not using the uniform contract standards that have been correlated on a national basis with previously determined outcomes. Instead, they often use very general guidelines that have not been verified from a medical-scientific or medical-legal standpoint. They are, in short, a throwback to the outdated community standard of practice and are counterproductive to any national cost and quality control effort.[11]

Although the best medical technology, which forms the basis for medical standards, is available, it is not being utilized effectively for the purchasers' benefit. There are several major reasons for this:

A serious lack of uniformity in the application of medical standards that have already been validated and accepted by the appropriate boards and bodies. This has resulted in wide disparities in quality of care among consumers, locations, and hospitals.

Enormous delays in getting new, already validated and accepted standards out to the community hospitals and implemented. Unlike a new engineering standard, it normally takes a new medical standard at least four or five years, and as much as twenty years, to be disseminated across the country.

A noticeable lack of backup systems in the hospital, where 85 to 90 percent of preventable damage occurs, to catch human error. Incompetence is rarely a factor—many backup systems are part of one or more standards, but are simply not enforced.

A lack of awareness on the part of hospitals and their staffs of what standards they should be holding themselves to. In instances of "defensive medicine" a standard or its standard criteria will not be followed and other superfluous services, such as tests or x-rays, will be performed. If an adverse outcome results and legal action is taken by the consumer, the additional services are totally nonadmissable since they do not relate to the contract standard. Unfortunately, the courts and the settlement process have been the continuing medical-legal education for providers: only when an adverse outcome occurs does the provider learn what standards he was required to maintain.

This process will continue indefinitely until purchasers have a loss control system assuring that all standards are applied uniformly, that new standards are disseminated and implemented as rapidly as possible, and that hospital backup systems are in operation. Only then can an acceptable return on investment be realized.[12]

Furthermore, the loss control system must have medical-legal as well as medical-scientific validity. If the standards that the suppliers agree to under the benefits contract are not maintained, the purchaser must have options available in the form of legal and economic sanctions. The purchaser should have an independent, forensically based monitoring-auditing system operating in his behalf to provide these options and to assure effective loss control while maximizing outcomes.

The question should be asked, "What is the provider required to give the purchaser?" Health services should be subject to contract law like any other service or product in our economy. Traditionally, purchasers have used the concept of contract law in the purchase of benefits only in very general terms. A contract with a third-party insurance carrier has, for example, covered hospitalization up to 120 days or a predetermined number of surgical procedures. The purchasers, however, have not specified, as is done in industry, what the outcomes of these services shall be in terms of nationally accepted medical-scientific standards that have been revalidated in the courts as medical-legal standards. However, as purchasers begin to document the massive drain on their budgets and the adverse impact on health of inadequate services, they will insist as a condition of the benefit contract that all standards be followed.

As a foundation for the development of these necessary contract standards, a group of concepts have been scrutinized.[13] The meaning of a standard from a legal tort point of view and from a contract point of view has been reasonably well documented.[14] From the medical-scientific standpoint, a number of publications have collated a specific "standard" in a variety of medical specialty fields.[15] The subject of clinical medical standardization has been addressed by the American Medical Association and the American Hospital Association in various position papers and other documents.[16] Methods of examination of standards from the standpoint of proximal causation of adverse outcomes and their prevention have been documented and utilized,[17] and finally, standards assessment for the protection of limited medical resources from a societal standpoint has also been done.[18]

These general medical and scientific principles that have been recognized in both common and codified law provide a basis for my collation of eight laws of medical standards. The first states that the most usually accepted standard is that which will produce the least amount of preventable death and/or disease, statistically and actuarially. This law comes from common negligence laws. There are four elements of negligence, all of which must be present to determine a finding of negligence: duty, dereliction, direct cause, and damage.

The best way to ascertain "duty" is to determine what the provider is holding himself out to give. This is usually encompassed in the first law of medical standards. Conversely, in order for a standard to be judged effective, its absence must produce damage statistically and actuarially. Otherwise, we have no criterion of the efficacy of a standard from the standpoint of the first law. From a benefit standpoint, the purchaser should buy only those services that are known to minimize damage and thus minimize death and/or disease statistically and actuarially. Therefore, if the provider on any given occasion states that "x process is not really necessary," then it becomes the right of the purchaser to refuse payment for that process. In short, the first law of medical standards encompasses the common principles of both law and medicine. It deals strictly in probability of events' occurring and requires proof of those probabilities that is adequately, scientifically documented.

The second law of medical standards is a corollary of the first: the accepted standard is that which will produce the least amount of preventable death and/or disease, or conversely, the greatest number of years of life and/or working days at the lowest possible cost. In comparing two processes that lead to the same outcome, the process that costs less must be used.

The third law of medical standards is that a standard must have a specifically defined clinical efficacy, with the least number of false positives, the least number of false negatives, and the greatest amount of direct correlation with desired outcome. The fourth law states that a medical standard and its efficacy are determined by the capability of specific backup systems, and that their capabilities must be determined by the doctrines of "reasonable man," "last clear chance of prevention," and the "contract standard of practice."

The fifth law is that a medical standard must have a specific return on investment, particularly in terms of protecting a set amount of resources for medical expenditure. This return on investment must be in terms of years of life and/or working days, and in terms of net benefit to society. The sixth law states that the individual to whom the medical standard is to be applied must be fully informed in terms he can understand so that its effects may permit him to live in the manner of his choosing. The seventh law of medical standards states that there must be the right to buy and to utilize any or all the services or processes designated as medical standards in accordance with the sixth law. The eighth law of medical standards states that the individual has the right to delegate the buying power to an agent acting in his behalf.

In order to assure that uniform standard criteria are used by providers, according to the laws of medical standards, an independent national system to monitor all services must be developed. This system would assure that every child's tonsilectomy is performed under circumstances that produce the best benefit-to-risk ratio, that women in hospitals will have a greatly reduced complication rate from pregnancy and delivery, that neonatal mental retardation will be minimized, and that the frequency and, more importantly, the severity of postoperative infection will be decreased. Uniform standard criteria would have a direct and measurable effect, therefore, in reducing required health services and, at the same time, in reducing the spillover effects on sick pay, disability benefits, Workmen's Compensation, death benefits, absenteeism, cost of retraining, and cost of rehabilitation.

Damm and Associates has become increasingly aware of the need for purchasers to develop these contract standards so that they will have the pragmatic tools to assure the best outcomes for their health dollars. Initial discussions with several major purchasers resulted in an expressed interst in attacking this seemingly unsolvable dilemma. Operating as the official claims review monitoring agent under the Federal Privacy Act of 1974, Damm and Associates has been working for a group of these major corporations over the last year to develop retrieval systems of valid patient utilization data from their carriers and their hospital. These systems have enabled the corporations to obtain valid data on hospital patient discharges which has never before been acquired. This has been in statistical summary form; no individual patient data was ever furnished to the employer.

The system also permits determination of disparities by employee location in cost of services and frequency of services compared with national contract standards, and of the extent of errors and omissions through comparison of the medical records and the related claims data used as justification for payment by the carriers. It has also developed options for expanding retrieval capabilities with a national system for monitoring inpatient discharges and for comparing services received with national contract standards. A users' group has been established by agreement among the corporations to share data and discuss ideas for additional cooperation. Finally, the system provides the basis for a loss control system for health services with a measured return on investment.

The results of these activities were very revealing and most encouraging. Of the claims data requested from insurance carriers, 100 percent was furnished, and over 75 percent of the medical records requested from hospitals were retrieved. After the initial precedents for retrieving data were established, claims data were eventually furnished within a two-week period and medical records within a three-week period. This supports the feasibility of developing a monitoring system to collect data on a national basis. Analysis of the claims and medical record data indicated a variety of opportunity areas, such as abnormally high complication rates in pregnancy, high frequencies of adverse risk-to-benefit surgeries, and significant disparities in hospital charges. This would justify the retrieval of data on a national basis to achieve the necessary statistical validity for all services. An unusually high error and ommission rate in the medical records was determined, which emphasizes the critical need for an independent monitoring system.

The extent of unnecessary and preventable costs and damage revealed by these data indicates that the return on investment from a loss control program would be substantial. TRW, Inc., has estimated that the amount saved by the reduction of the highest risk-to-benefit surgery alone would cover the cost of the entire program in the first year of implementation. It is projected overall that a conservative return on investment from a total loss control program including carrier and hospital charges and employee-consumer education would approximate a factor of three to five in the first year, and five to seven in the second year of implementation, depending upon the purchaser's objectives.

The establishment of the system's data base has already begun with the basic research and documentation on preventable and unnecessary costs and damage, and the data retrieval prototypes designed and implemented for Damm and Associates' clients. There are some commonalities among all employee populations, but marked epidemiological differences exist based on such factors as type of industry, age, sex, and location. Therefore, the tailored design of each purchaser's data base is critical. The next step is to begin full monitoring of the hospitals serving the largest employee locations, in order to increase the validity of these purchasers' data bases. At the same time, the inclusion of additional purchasers from industry, labor, and government will allow the identification of additional opportunity areas.

The data are retrieved from medical monitoring forms placed in selected hospitals by the carriers. These are accompanied by patient release forms designed in accordance with the Federal Privacy Act of 1974. The monitoring forms are filled out by the hospital's medical records department on every discharged employee and dependent. They contain critical data that would indicate a deviation or a high probability of deviation from contract standards in known risk areas. These data points are compared with a medical standards data bank to reflect the degree of deviation. The patient data is correlated with spillover data on, for example, disability benefits, to determine related opportunity areas. This is used as an ongoing measurement to indicate the effectiveness of the program in reducing cost and increasing quality. The standards data bank is constantly updated to reflect the latest additions or modifications in medical-scientific and medical-legal standards.

Reports with statistical summary data are furnished to the purchasers on a regular basis, continually presenting the areas of greatest opportunity and providing options for loss control program development and implementation. Collated reports covering two or more purchasers are provided to those purchasers who have entered into separate agreements to share summary data. The users' group provides an ongoing forum for sharing data and for joint discussion of loss control efforts on a local or national basis.

A developed, statistically valid data base for all selected employee locations allows the purchaser to begin precertification of those opportunity areas selected for loss control activities. Precertification is a review process whereby all diagnostic and therapeutic procedures are screened against standards or standard criteria that have already been validated and adopted by providers. Approximately 90 to 95 percent of all procedures can be precertified in this manner. Precertification forms, designed and reviewed by a national advisory committee, are distributed to the hospitals by the carriers. These forms are incorporated into both the preadmission process and selected departments, such as obstetrics, that have indicated the highest opportunity areas for recouping cost. For example, when an employee is to be precertified for a given surgery, only those tests indicated are given and the results are compared against the standard criteria for either indication or contraindication. This process eliminates the need for a second opinion except in those cases where the physician disagrees either with the standard criteria or the diagnostic results. In that case, the physician supplies dissenting documentation which is then reviewed by an advisory committee. In all instances, the patient is fully informed fo the standard criteria being used and of any dissenting opinions.

This precertification process creates an "insurance program" for the hospital and the medical staff. With procedures following nationally accepted standards, the risk of malpractice action is either eliminated or greatly reduced. This process can be used to correlate malpractice insurance premiums for both hospitals and medical staffs with the degree of precertification utilization. In addition, the precertification data is added to the data base to be compared with the data from the medical monitoring forms. This provides a way to minimize the system's error rate and to increase the effectiveness of all forms.

The theoretical underpinnings for such a national system have been adequately documented. Now it is time for the purchasers of services to join together in developing a national data base through constant monitoring to identify the nature and extent of loss control opportunities. The system assures the delivery of services that produce predictable outcomes as predetermined by the purchasers of health services. Only those services that produce the best outcomes should be included in any benefit plan for employees and their families. This is an item for cooperation between labor and government, employee and employer, public and private sector, and should be viewed as a "benefit" to assure the best outcomes of all benefits.

NOTES

1. "The Skyrocketing Costs of Health Care," *Business Week*, May 17, 1976.

2. *HEW Administration of the Professional Standards Review Organization (PSRO) Program*, Hearing before the Subcommittee on Oversight of the Committee on Ways and Means, U.S. House of Representatives, May 21, 1976; and Ralph Emerson, M.D., "Unjustified Surgery: Fact or Myth?" *New York State Journal of Medicine*, March 1976.

3. Loring W. Wood, M.D., "The Bronx Study: A Trial of Health Care Management," *Journal of Occupational Medicine*, vol. 17, October 1975.

4. Ibid.

5. Prior literature documentation analyses of over 1,000 professional and medical product liability case summaries from the United States, Japan, Canada, and Great Britain, from the Damm and Associates data bank, 1970–1977; "Ribicoff Commission," "Medical Malpractice: The Patient vs. the Physician," Study submitted by the Subcommittee on Executive Reorganization to the Committee on Government Operations, November 1969; Leon S. Pocincki, et al., "The Incidence of Iatrogenic Injuries," Report of the Secretary's Commission on Medical Malpractice, Depart-

ment of Health, Education, and Welfare, Washington, D.C., January 1973; Ribicoff, op cit.; National Association of Insurance Commissioners, *Malpractice Claims,* vol. 1, no. 1, December 1975.

6. Alain C. Enthoven, "National Health Insurance and the Cost of Medical Care," Address to the Detroit Academy of Medicine, May 13, 1975.

7. National Association of Insurance Commissioners, op cit.; National Association of Insurance Commissioners, *Malpractice Claims,* vol. 1, no. 2, April 1976, vol. 1, no. 3, September 1976 and vol. 1, no. 4, June 1977.

8. Ribicoff, op cit.

9. Henry C. Damm, "Health Cost and Quality Control: A Medical-Legal Approach," Address to the Employee Health Forum at Case Western Reserve University, March 22, 1976.

10. Thomas H. Ainsworth, Jr., M.D., *Quality Assurance Program for Medical Care in the Hospital,* American Hospital Association, 1972.

11. Subcommittee on Oversight of the Committee on Ways and Means, op cit.

12. Karl Bunkelman, "A Medical-Legal Health Cost and Quality Approach for the Industrial Community," Health Resource Center, May 1976.

13. Emerson, op cit.

14. William L. Prosser, *Handbook of the Law of Torts,* 4th ed. (St. Paul: West Publishing, 1971); and Arthur Linton Corbin, *Corbin on Contracts* (St. Paul: West Publishing, 1963).

15. Henry C. Damm, *The Practical Manual for Clinical Laboratory Procedures* (Cleveland: Chemical Rubber Co., 1976); and Henry C. Damm, *Handbook of Clinical Laboratory Data* (Cleveland: Chemical Rubber Co., 1965).

16. Bruce A. Flasher, et al., "Professional Standards Review Organization," Journal of the American Medical Association, vol. 233, no. 13, 1973; AMA Center for Health Services, Research and Development, AMA Division of Medical Practice, November 1970, and the AMA Department of Environmental, Public and Occupational Health, (Division of Scientific Activities), January 1971, *Information Papers,* AMA, 1971; and Ainsworth, op cit.

17. Secretary's Commission on Medical Malpractice, op cit; Morris Crawford, "Response to Subcommittee—Medical Malpractice: the Patient vs. the Physician," Study submitted by the Subcommittee on Government Operations, U.S. Senate, 1969; and Prior literature documentation analyses of over 1,000 professional and medical product liability case summaries from the United States, Japan, Canada, and Great Britain, from the Damm and Associates data bank, 1970–1977.

18. Howard A. Hiatt, "Protecting the Medical Commons: Who is Responsible?" *New England Journal of Medicine,* 293:235–241, July 1975.

CHALLENGES

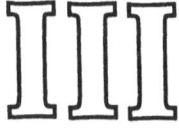

Corporate Reaction to the Occupational Safety and Health Act of 1970

Karl T. Benedict, Sr.

14

The Occupational Safety and Health Act of 1970 has already had its initial impact on corporate health clinics. Much more is to come, however, as criteria develop and regulations become refined scientifically and legally. Balanced judgments and economic feasibility are critical to the entire environmental health effort, not only in the United States but worldwide. The effect of OSHAct to date on all industries and occupations covered has been quite variable as the regulations and the act itself have wound their tedious way through a maze of interpretations, compliances, inspections, variances, and legal wrangles until finally, six years after its passage, the Supreme Court declared OSHAct constitutional. No doubt some industries fighting the act hoped for the same course of events that killed the National Recovery Act of Franklin D. Roosevelt's day.

Whether these legal procedures were intended to nullify the act or any part thereof, they continue and, in truth, have delayed implementation of many of its provisions while forcing the cabinet secretary responsible for enforcement to revise administrative procedures, modify and delay regulations, and conduct prolonged hearings. Labor has been impatient; industries, confused; and corporate medical clinics have had to mark time or proceed on self-determined courses.

Yet, despite the resistance of industry, few would dare to disagree with the idealism or intent of the act—that is, to require employers to furnish their employees a safe and healthful workplace. Indeed, such goals are hardly even new: the situation leading to the act has been recognized ever since the ancient Greeks realized that certain dusts and metals were health hazards to artisans and miners. The sagas of injuries to agricultural workers undoubtedly predate written records. The dangers of being stepped on by an elephant or gored by a water buffalo must have been described by grandfather to father and father to son for centuries. There were no first aid or health clinics available for these workers. Nor were there any OSHA forms 100, 101, or 102 for their employers to complete.

Nowadays, the cause and prevention of industrial accidents is better understood than those of occupational diseases, carcinogenesis, and genetic defects. Hence, OSHA undertook to attack the accident problem first. Industrial, legal, safety, and government organizations became embroiled in so-called nit-picking regulations, yet some may have prevented accidents. Some small employers were confused, dismayed, yet fined for violations. They sought exemption from the act. Some Congressmen agreed. Labor did not. Labor was critical of OSHA's delay in promulgating occupational disease standards. Whereas the accident prevention standards primarily concerned safety people, the impending occupational disease standards most certainly will affect the health clinic functions.

One must wonder why it took so long since Hippocrates and Galen recognized the relationship between work exposure and lead-induced disease, or since Sir Percival Pott described scrotal cancer resulting from chimney soot in young chimney sweeps in England, until the United States Congress wrote OSHAct in 1970. In the eighteenth century the Italian scientist, medical observer, and author, sometimes called the father of occupational medicine, Bernard Ramazzini, described forty-two occupations with observable ill effects in his book *De Morbis Artificium Diatriba* and subsequent writing. He also included possible protective measures. Miners, chemists, glass workers, stone cutters, printers, and weavers were listed. This exceeds OSHA's first list of target industries. He even included tobacco workers and corpse bearers. Obviously, OSHA's regulations are more comprehensive and scientifically more accurate and they do define with varying specificity health clinic procedures.

One must wonder why so many problems plague OSHA progress given the long history of the developing knowledge of occupational diseases. Furthermore, why can industry, labor, government, and the health professions not get together more effectively to eliminate the more serious, more obvious, and more extensive occupational diseases first. Yet, as recently as 1975, Powell and Christensen explained that delay in the development of criteria was due in part to lack of sufficient literature and research data. In the meantime, health costs continue to rise. Witness the effect of coal miners' black lung disease on the

Social Security system. How much less literature and data were available to Hippocrates and Ramazzini!

Literature concerned with health problems of workmen increased during the nineteenth century; likewise, legislation was significantly broadened. There were the coal mining acts, a factory act, cotton cloth factory acts, and so on in England. Workmen's compensation for industrial injuries existed in Germany in 1844, but not in the United States until seventy-five years later. Between 1910 and 1912 the Bureau of Mines was created; New York passed its Workmen's Compensation law and both New York and California had compulsory reporting of occupational diseases; Harvard University and the Massachusetts Institute of Technology established a course in public health; the National Safety Council was set up; the first American Congress on Industrial Diseases was held; Dr. Alice Hamilton published her studies on lead poisoning; and L. J. Hams of the New York City Department of Health reported on mercurialism in the hat industry.

In 1914 chest x-rays were first used by Lanza and Higgins to study pulmonary diseases in Missouri miners. In 1916 Congress enacted a model Workmen's Compensation law for civilian employees in the United States (Mississippi was the last state to enact such a law in 1948). In 1929 safe limits for dust in granite cutting plants were established, and were in part the basis for the current OSHA silica standard for this target industry. Yet as recently as during the Industrial Hygiene Foundation Silica Symposium of 1975, this standard was challenged.

Prior to safety and Workmen's Compensation legislation, ill-trained, uneducated, and especially foreign workers suffered amputated limbs, crushed skulls, and broken backs. The injured worker was tossed on the scrap heap of lost souls or buried without ceremony; common law offered little aid to him or his family. Lack of finances, education, and legal aid plus the two common legal defenses, "assumption of risk" and "contributory negligence," nullified many claims. Courts and legislatures sought to solve this problem by enacting the Employer's Liability Act transferring the assumption of risk from the employer to an insurance carrier. However, the latter could often evade the law because the claimant could not prove the employer at fault or negligent.

For instance, according to Rutherford J. Johnston, 235 men were killed in Allegheny County, Pennsylvania, in one year, yet 54 per cent of their families received no Workmen's Compensation benefits. In Cuyahoga County, Ohio, in ten years only 36 percent of the deaths were compensated—at an average of $838.61 each.

Data on the development of Workmen's Compensation laws in the United States vary in many textbooks because only partial information is given or such data are used in reference to a particular subject. Carl E. Geuther wrote that acts in several states, beginning with an elective act in Maryland, were declared unconstitutional. The Wisconsin act of 1911 was the first to survive. James A. Tobey wrote that the first comprehensive act was passed in New York in 1910 and upheld by the United States Supreme Court in 1916. Washington state enacted a law in 1911. In 1920 only six states, California, Connecticut, Hawaii, Massachusetts, North Dakota, and Wisconsin, provided compensation for occupational diseases, while only twenty-five states covered occupational diseases by 1943, according to W. C. Dreessen.

With these laws came new legal terminology such as "industrial accidents," "personal injury," "arising out of," and "in the course of." These would seem simple, yet varying court opinions filled a two-volume law treatise by Arthur Larson. Obviously, Workmen's Compensation costs rose and plagued business people. Countermeasures were adopted: improved safety, better care of injured workers, industrial hygeine surveys and controls, preemployment and periodic examinations, and special placement studies. Health and radiation physicists, medical secretaries and technicians, and consultant specialists joined the team of the loss prevention organization. Thus were born the corporate occupational health services of today.

My survey of Norton's medium-sized clinic revealed one new industrial injury case for every thirty visits. Seven were for retreatment of a previous accident and twenty-two were for examinations and medical problems. One should not conclude, however, that this cinic was moving into private medical care like an HMO. The ratio of initial visits to retreatments was one to four. If the condition was serious, the employee was referred to his physician. On return, he was rechecked for his ability to undertake his particular duties. Only minor, nondisabling conditions were treated. Preventive measures were limited to tetanus injections for any employee, injections for overseas travelers on company business, limited checkup on persons with controllable medical problems, and certain educational programs.

Because Workmen's Compensation laws and benefits vary greatly from state to state, OSHA has been developing recommendations for upgrading and standardizing them. The past variations in coverage were industrial accidents only versus industrial accidents and specified occupational diseases. The state legislature—not a physician—might determine that one worker, ill because of exposure to silica-bearing dust, deserved compensation whereas a fellow worker had noncompensable beryllium lung disease. One state had separate industrial accident and occupational disease laws. Even Massachusetts, with one of the most comprehensive, labor-oriented laws, had a top limit for silicosis compensation benefits about one-third the benefit level for industrial accidents. There was possibly a justifiable reason at the time. The philosophy of Workmen's Compensation had two phases: compensation, and rehabilitation to gainful, taxpaying employment. This latter program rose after World War I as disabled veterans sought work, and fell as business went down and formerly scarce labor became overabundant.

The latest federal and state rehabilitation regulations parallel the OSHA regulations in their impact on corporate clinics. Likewise, heart-stroke-cancer from smoking, alcoholism, and diabetes educational campaigns are impacting heavily, if voluntarily, on corporate clinics. Obviously, therefore, corporate health care clinics develop under the influence of state safety, health, and labor laws, Workmen's Compensation decisions and costs, labor union pressure, the kind of industry, and the availability of community health services. Lack of the latter resulted in the initiation of the Kaiser Plan and Foundation, the basis for the HMO concept.

Nevertheless, many of these developments are not new. One should read *Health Services in Industry* by my predecessor and teacher at Norton Company from 1911 to 1948, W. I. Clark, and particularly note his listed functions of an industrial health department. His title was service director and his responsibilities included everything from safety to sanitation, from restaurant service to welfare and even banking (employee credit union). The Norton Clinic, established in 1911, included a central dispensary, three satellite first aid clinics, an x-ray department, twenty-two nurses, two full-time physicians, four part-time physician specialists, and a medical secretary. Records were maintained from the beginning noting all clinic visits. In 1943, for instance, 160,000 clinic visits were noted for approximately 9,000 employees working in a heavy, sometimes hot, sometimes dusty, overtime, wartime environment. Today, certain laboratory and special eye and heart tests have been added. Pulmonary function testing has been done for over twenty years with ever-improving equipment. Yet, more can be done. Management constantly reviews its programs with all personnel departments and upgrades them. Currently, it runs antismoking campaigns, cancer education programs, and free blood pressure clinics—none of this required by OSHA or government regulations.

Corporate health care was a part of the field of industrial medicine in 1922. To illustrate, in one factory employing 3,600 people there were two reportable contagious disease epidemics in four years. There were seventy-three cases of mumps, twenty-seven cases of German measles, and one case of smallpox. However, during the 1918–1919 influenza epidemic, the onset of illness was so violent and death occurred so rapidly that this company set aside an emergency first aid unit and morgue in case someone died at work. Little wonder then that older persons and companies were willing to run the risk of swine flu vaccinations.

"The Cardiac in Industry" was the title of a presentation by Dr. E. W. Robertson in 1920. The x-ray was used to diagnose occupational pulmonary disease, tuberculosis, and fractures. Examination of middle-aged men was recommended to detect degenerative diseases early enough to arrest their progress. Why then are some persons and some industries so critical of the health care functions outlined in OSHA regulations? Why should some groups want to prevent preplacement examinations? Why should some object to classification of worker health status into grades A, B, C, or D? These things should be done to protect the employee and our society. Had they been done voluntarily, OSHA regulations would not have been necessary. To quote Dr. Clark again: "To simply reject a man with active tuberculosis without telling him of his condition and advising him what to do is a social crime exposing others to the disease and preventing the possible cure of the affected man."

However, there may be reasons to consider and possibly question the impact of OSHA on corporate health care. First, any new government program or regulation involves educational programs, new procedures, and variable amounts of time, paperwork, and storage space. This reduces profits and funds available for employee benefits. Second, there is fear of interference with privacy of information about processes, products, wages, and fringe benefits. Third, such interference may lead to leakage of information or trade secrets to competitors. Fourth, this might disclose illegal operations, unsafe practices, or unhealthy conditions like the Gauley Bridge episode. Fifth, criticism of operations, correctly or not, can produce adverse psychological effects on management or labor. Sixth, the complexities of OSHA regulations have obviously led to many challenges and legal battles such as those cases going to the United States Supreme Court recently. These are terribly time-consuming and costly to small employers. And seventh, the health clinics of small and medium-sized employers must seek outside consultant assistance which is often not available. To illustrate, many small communities and one-industry towns do not have readily available toxicological or otological consultant services. They might have to cease operations. The doctor shortage is greatest in rural areas; full-time and even part-time trained occupational health personnel, and particularly doctors, are often not available.

Large industries can comply and probably should comply fully with OSHA regulations. Compliance has changed the format of the medical program in my company from comprehensive, general medical examinations and limited treatments to more frequent, limited, yet more intense studies of certain persons in high-risk jobs identified by OSHA in new regulations. New laboratory procedures in-plant or outside will be required as new chemicals and related regulations are introduced. There will be increased costs in equipment, record-keeping, and personnel. OSHA has had some impact on corporate health care already, but much more must be anticipated now that the Supreme Court has declared the act constitutional and entry without a warrant is legal— as it has been in Massachusetts since 1877.

Compliance with new standards for solvents, chemicals, or materials that produce dusts, vapors, or fumes can prove to be an expensive process. Each standard will contain seven basic sections: environmental; medical surveillance; labeling; personal protective equipment and clothing; employee appraisal, instruction, and education; work practices; and sanitation practices, lockers, clothing, and so on.

Besides the news reports of illnesses and deaths of persons exposed to asbestos, kepone, PCB, BCME, vinyl chloride, and other carcinogens and mutagenic substances, the "Toxic Substance List" with over 25,000 entries prepared by NIOSH in 1974 led, by title alone, to opportunities for legal action against companies never anticipated by NIOSH or the industries. Accordingly, the 1975 edition is entitled "Registry of Toxic Effects of Chemical Substances." It added 4,000 new compounds and gives information on 1,545 carcinogens, 30 involving mutagenesis, 250 involving teratogenesis, and 700 with definite human effects. Since then, medical surveillance involves preplacement, periodic, and special examinations according either to the general duty clause or to specific standards; special screening procedures, tests, and x-rays; and accurate record maintenance and retention for specified intervals.

The impact is specific for the exposure involved in named industries. A data source for in-plant research and governmental epidemiological studies is to be created, not only to rule in, but to rule out industrial exposures per se. Furthermore, the facilities (personnel, equipment, and location) and organization make medical surveillance units in large corporate health clinics feasible and adaptable to improving community ambulatory health care. In smaller communities, it can be the backbone of this care; in large communities; it can be a major component of total health care, especially since many hospitals and large clinics of HMOs are not prepared to practice this kind of preventive health maintenance. Most noncorporate physicians are primarily concerned with general medical diagnosis and therapy, with rare interest in the environmental etiology of diseases. (This may change rapidly as HEW hospital curtailments increase.)

There are four major factors that could assist progress toward OSHA goals. One is political change. President Ford was going to make major changes. Now, President Carter plans to make other changes. However, changing the HEW secretary and agency staff as often as has been done in OSHA and NIOSH certainly delays implementation of any new programs. A second factor is labor or business pressures. The soundness of these segments of our economy are very critical at times like depression and war. Survival supersedes ideal health programs. A third is uncontrolled or foreign influences: war, cold war, energy. The latter could lead to economic reverses and abandonment or marked curtailment of many ideal programs such as those of OSHA, NIOSH, NIH, EPA, or EEO, all of which involve corporate health. Finally, legal-judicial decisions could be a major factor.

The Problems of Industry-Sponsored Health Programs

Sheldon W. Samuels

15

The revolution in values in our society, symbolized by clusters of concepts often labeled "environment" and "participation," creates expectations that did not exist only a few years ago. It is in this context that we must view the opinions said to be commonly held by workers regarding physicians and surgeons in the employ of industry ("company doctors"). Although they may have been long held, these opinions form the basis of an emerging crisis. The threshold for the acceptance or rejection of existing medical care related to the workplace has been altered radically by this revolution.

Note the careful statement, "opinions *said* to be commonly held by workers." There is very little developed information on what rank-and-file workers think about company doctors. There is, however, a preliminary study by the Industrial Union Department of the AFL-CIO that may characterize the problem.[1]

A Crisis in Confidence

There is little question in my mind about what most elected union officials think of company doctors and the company doctor system,* and the data in the above-cited study indicate that the views of union leaders closely reflect membership opinions. There are at least five views currently held. The first and most essential is that company doctors are no less a part of management than the plant engineer, personnel director, or the chairman of the board. They are seen as tools of the boss. My personal opinion, molded in part by research and in part by wishful thinking, is that some elements of an acceptable patient-physician relationship may often exist. Certainly, there is often a reciprocal desire for this to be true. Unfortunately, attitudes are formed less by ideals than by functional and economically defined peer groups. In other words, the plant situation breeds attitudes inimical to the development of a "normal" patient-physician relationship.

These attitudes are reinforced by easily discovered legal and historical factors. A company doctor is not legally responsible for malpractice—the company is. In some states, such as New Jersey, workers may not even recover damages from an employer for such wrongdoing except when it is intentional. There is no legal reason for most industrial physicians to be responsive to the needs of workers. Historically, in addition, the company doctor has failed to achieve the same degree of self-regulation and institutional protection from exploitation that prevails in the other branches of medicine.** Most important, he has failed—at least publicly—to establish common cause with the worker on key issues in the plant, in the community, or in the legislature.† On the contrary, the company doctor is seen defending the corporate interests or playing out a role characterized by a Nuremberg silence on key issues. It is too often the case that the company physician or surgeon finds no ethical reason to be responsive to the needs of workers,‡ and the professional structures of industrial medicine mirror this weakness.

A second view is that the company doctor, even if it is his wish, often cannot protect the confidentiality of his patient's records or even share records that the worker considers his own. In a dispute between the United Mine

*I meet on a quarterly basis with presidents, secretary-treasurers, and vice-presidents of international unions representing a cross section of affiliates of the AFL-CIO. This topic is frequently discussed.

**The American Occupational Medical Association has adopted a code of ethics only within the last year and is still discussing a means of implementation. The effectiveness of voluntary efforts of this kind has yet to be demonstrated. This pessimism has been reinforced by the failure of AOMA (or the AMA) to investigate publicized cases of alleged malpractice in Indianapolis, Joplin, Vernon (California), Pascagoula, Roanoke, Houston, Kellogg, Tacoma, Pottstown, Hopewell, Tyler, Port Allegheny, and other communities.

†It may be unfair to single out the company doctor on this issue. Recently, the Pennsylvania Thoracic Society refused to become involved in setting up a system of surveillance for a high-risk group (asbestos) of workers in Port Allegheny, Pennsylvania, on the grounds that such involvement might stir controversy.

‡The first principle of any ethical system must be the biblical injunction to choose life. This is a basic principle from which all others emanate, including those moral dicta called rights, and without which no human society could or should survive. A worker's right to know of the danger to

Workers and Bethlehem Steel, the arbitrator—a physician— took the position that doctors employed by the company have a conflict of interest that would not be acceptable in other sectors. Moreover, he noted a "legacy of distrust" based on the reality of broken confidentiality that had led to discriminatory treatment of workers. The access of workers to their medical records was won by a 1969 strike against the Johns-Manville plant in Manville, New Jersey, in which such access was one issue. In a similar situation in 1973, the labor movement called a national boycott against Shell.

A third view is that a company medical program, like any other component of corporate structure, must justify itself by either long-term or short-term dollar benefits. Doctors in this position are less likely to be on the worker's side in Workmen's Compensation cases, definition of environmental conditions affecting health, the impact of the plant on community resources, or the interpretation of preemployment and other medical examinations required by the Occupational Safety and Health Act (OSHAct). Even when he is, his position in the company is not usually influential enough to balance the arguments of other department heads.

A fourth view is that in-plant medical care is poor in quality and quantity. Most workers are not covered by company medical programs and most of those covered receive little systematic attention. Certainly, with few exceptions, they receive nothing like executive medical programs. Even among companies with 50,000 or more employees, 19 percent of the firms have no full-time physician and of those that do, only 35 percent of the employees have access to him. Among all these companies, 60 percent of the employees have no access to either a full- or part-time physician or nurse.[2]

Finally, there is growing difficulty in accepting plant programs as resources unrelatable and separate from the total medical care delivery system. None of this is new. Workers may have had these feelings since the beginning of the industrial revolution. What is new is the new worker.

The New Worker

The worker's new perception of his environment is accompanied by a strengthened will to participate fully in the decisions that affect his life in every sphere and at every stage of his effort to achieve a better life. This is a conception of life formed by the dramatic changes in the value systems among workers of this generation. A primary effect of the eight-hour workday and better-than-subsistence wages has been the leisure and financial ability to absorb information made available by mass communications, mass education,

---

which he is exposed derives from his need to know. This and all rights arise from the need to preserve life.

The relevance of this to real life is seen in the examination of industrial practice. A paper in Chemistry and Industry by a Dr. Gadian, medical officer of Lankro Chemicals, on the control of alpha napthylamine in the past decade outlined the following procedure: assume a latency period of at least eighteen years for bladder cancer, hire a man over forty, and play God—assume that it is quite all right if he dies at age fifty-eight.

This and similar approaches are frequent proposals, if not practices. The fact is that the industrial physician often does not choose life—quite the opposite.

and a broadened sphere of day-to-day personal contacts. No longer isolated by language or limited by the capacity of his ethnic institutions for social and political action (as was his father), the modern industrial worker is in a position to examine the quality of his life and to effect change directly, through his union, and by his personal involvement in the decision-making processes of myriad social and political structures.

The consequence has been that millions of workers have rejected the blind continuation of their subsidy of the environment of the workplace. The result: a bitter two-year battle that culminated in 1970 in OSHAct. This stringent legislation sets forth relatively new and expanded rights for workers, which, while they have evolved from need, concomitantly reflect workers' environmental concern and their will to participate in its expression.

Participatory rights, as a widespread and widely accepted principle of our society, developed relatively late in Western political thought; "liberty," "civil rights," and other issues and overlapping concepts clearly predate "participation." Participatory rights have largely developed in our time in response to broader needs in the community, where the demand to take part in public hearings, be heard at school board meetings, and become involved through similar points of entry in the political system has been overwhelming. The new set of participatory rights includes those demanded by the worker during the hearings held in conjunction with the passage of OSHAct through Congress. The legislative history of the act establishes that many of these rights were not preconceived by union or congressional staff. In a heartening demonstration of the "system" at its best, they actually came from the rank and file. Unfortunately, it is only now—six years after passage of the act—that there is any hope that these provisions can be fully implemented. But even the partial implementation of the act in its early years has stimulated a massive, positive involvement by the nation's work force.

An Alternative System

The conventional problems faced by the medical community—training, services, facilities, and personnel—will continue to be aggravated by the OSHAct as its impact unfolds. Moreover, the rediscovery of bystander and family effects of occupational exposure is enlarging the scope of occupational disease treatment. Without question, the total community health care delivery system must be expanded to treat work place, bystander, and family effects or it will collapse. The adequacy of our response will be determined by the extent to which we take into account the participatory factor—it is a dimension that cannot be neglected. This is clear in the apparent rejection of the existing system of industrial medical services.

Prior to the passage of the act, workers bargained—sometimes with success—for separation of the doctor or nurse from management, for better and more comprehensive services, for confidentiality, for access to medical records, and for free choice of physician. Some of these issues have been decided by the act and will be subsumed under the standard-setting provisions. Access to medical records has been established (but largely unimplemented to date) and specific medical services are being mandated, but other issues will be in contention for some time. During that time, judging by the current pattern, labor's demands will be overwhelmingly participatory in character. Medical decisions, in labor's view, can no longer be a matter between the company and the company-employed doctor. The worker will need at least an equal voice. I predict aso that government will be given important roles in accreditation, record-keeping, and financial support.

The well-publicized controversies revolving around these issues in the black lung program, which covers fewer than 200,000 coal miners, will be dwarfed by similar issues involving some 57 million workers covered by the act and exposed for the first time to systematic information and education. Special brown lung (byssinosis) and white lung (asbestosis) programs already have been proposed. However, unlike the black lung program, I believe that the new programs will be integrated with broader community services, will have less dependence upon the federal government, and will draw upon the obligations of the employer and his insurance carrier for much of the funding. This can only mean profound changes in the quantity and character of these services and in industrial medicine in general.

One new program must inevitably be focused on the identification, notification, surveillance, and treatment of high-risk groups. Occupational disease has been established for centuries, but it was only with the passage of OSHAct in 1970 that significant progress has been made in identifying the large number of environmental agents associated with irreversible occupational disease. Predictions ridiculed and ignored for many years are being realized. Unless we achieve an amendment to the laws of nature, without preventive, preclinical, and clinical intervention, the biological implications of the past and current trends of essentially uncontrolled industrial production could mean widespread disaster.

For example, a well-defined carcinogenic process is coking. A number of coke oven emissions have been defined individually as cancer-producing; the current work population is known (30,000) as is the potentially exposed population (270,000 over forty-five years, assuming a 20 percent work-force turnover). Asbestos is also well-described in the literature. Currently, a million workers are heavily exposed to asbestos from clutch and brake lining maintenance alone. Another half-million are heavily exposed in mining, milling, fabrication, and construction. Most foreboding is the understanding that of the past one million asbestos-exposed shipyard workers, as many as 600,000 may develop asbestos-related disease.

In World War II some 400,000 workers were exposed to asbestos in the Brooklyn Navy Yard; 110,000 of these were heavily exposed. While no one knows the fate of these men and women, a seven-year study by Mount Sinai of 1,249 asbestos workers revealed the pattern we might expect: fifty-nine cases of lung cancer (of which fifty-seven are dead) and thirty-one cases of mesothelioma (of which thirty-one are dead). In this case, we have failed to intervene successfully because we do not know how. In most cases we fail to even try.

In Tyler, Texas, one high-risk group of workers, employed between 1954 and 1972 in an asbestos factory, has been placed under surveillance with serial observations by the East Texas Chest Hospital. The group has been identified and most members have been traced. Baseline clinical, radiological, and cytological studies are planned, but there is no reason to believe that what we know now will make any significant difference in the fate of the 850 individuals concerned. In any case, even alleviatory therapy is currently denied the workers. Most reviewers of the NCI-sponsored program consider the project a failure.

There is some evidence that approximately one-eighth of all deaths among groups of vinyl chloride polymerization workers will be of hepatic angiosarcoma, and that others among them may die in excess numbers of bronchogenic carcinoma, brain tumors, and lymphomas. Perhaps 30,000 such individuals are known to be at risk and, if incidence of neoplasms is found to be significantly increased among polyvinyl chloride fabrication workers, that number could grow to one million individuals exposed in the past. Our efforts at early diagnosis of hepatic angiosarcoma among vinyl chloride–exposed workers have failed. Neither available liver function tests nor radioisotope screening nor clinical examinations have allowed diagnosis of this fatal tumor early enough for intervention to have some chance of success.

In Louisville, Kentucky, large groups of current and former vinyl chloride polymerization workers have been brought under observation in an intensive study by the University of Louisville. Initial experience suggests that none of the available tools provides diagnosis of angiosarcoma or other neoplasms (lung, brain, lymphoma) early enough to allow hope for effective treatment. Reviewers of the project, which is also sponsored by NCI, are hopeful that new tools will evolve from this study.

These are a few examples of high-risk populations uncovered since the passage of OSHAct. There are at least 6 million additional workers, family members, and bystanders in defined high-risk populations, but there is no definable program of notification, surveillance, and clinical extension.

What is meant by a high-risk population is most easily shown by examples since it is a loosely defined concept. It is not possible to provide a meaningful estimate of the total number in all populations because of the lack of data, the continuous addition of new agents and processes to the "known" list, and the necessary assumption that large numbers of workers are in more than one population because of multiple exposure. Nevertheless it is fair to say that millions of people are at high risk and can be expected to die of cancer and other irreversible diseases at increasing rates proportional to the rate of the industrial development of the past forty-five years. But it is also fair to say that not everyone in a high-risk population will develop an environmentally related irreversible disease. Rates depend upon factors of individual biology and individual environment, such as heredity, duration of exposure, differences in the biological activities of the agents themselves or their metabolites, and the mode of exposure.

We have not created an apparatus in government or in the private sector aimed at reducing the risk of environmental exposure in the community and workplace through intervention. Some progress has been made in clinical research and the delivery of the therapeutic tools thus created, but these activities in most institutions are untied to environmental health and deal with disease essentially at the end of its development. What we are now faced with is the problem of filling in the gap. Even if effective, intervention usually will come too late to prevent the initiation of disease development for most members of high-risk groups. But the process must begin.

These gaps are difficult to close since they require enlightened and aggressive leadership to achieve a community of efforts necessary to overcome the instinct for administrative pettiness and organizational chauvinism that haunts large-scale operations. The time gap is most critical: we simply have not learned to address ourselves to the problem early enough. One of the most important concepts repeatedly established is the long period of clinical latency between onset of exposure (or, perhaps more accurately, "effective exposure") and clinical evidence of disease. This "silent period" between exposure and the discovery of disease is of more than theoretical interest. It offers an opportunity, a possibility—because of the delayed appearance implied—that intervention during this time might be successful in breaking the links between exposure to an agent and preclinical disease, between this stage and the development of early stages of clinical disease, and between these stages and uncontrollable disease. While there is no guarantee that it is certain or even likely to be the case, we should at least try to break at least some of the links in that chain of events. The fruitfulness of interrupting disease development is found in an estimate that we can expect 10,000 deaths from bladder cancer and that half these lives can be saved by existing methods of early detection.

The desperate need for an integrated industrial-community program aimed at early detection of preclinical disease receives scant attention. But such a program, either by itself or as part of a broader national health program, cannot be administered by the corporations that perpetuate the conditions from which the risk evolved. The conflict of interest and huge economic disincentive to a satisfactory relationship in which the worker—not the company—is the patient makes essential the element of participation by the worker in a noncorporate setting.

What I am proposing will necessitate an intimate integration of epidemiological, clinical, and laboratory approaches to occupational medicine at the community level outside the plant. Early recognition and understanding of these issues and their participatory characteristic should strengthen the ability of organized medicine to share effectively in the vital decisions that must be made. The doctor can no longer neglect the new dimension of health care taking form in the workplace.

NOTES

1. Sherry G. Sellivan and Ido de Groot, *Copperopolis Men, 1973,* Joint report of the University of Cincinnati and the Industrial Union Department of the AFL-CIO, 1973. See also Sheldon W. Samuels, "Lest We Forget," *Viewpoint,* vol. 3, no. 3, 1973.

2. Seymour Lusterman, *Industry Roles in Health Care* (New York: The Conference Board, 1974).

The Corporation and Its Environment: Corporate Responsibility in an Era of Limits

Rick J. Carlson

16

Marcos Vela had worked as a machine tender at the Johns-Manville asbestos plant in Pittsburgh, California, for 38 years. During those years he received a gold watch, two yearly dinners, and two lungfuls of dust. Vela has advanced pneumoconiosis—commonly known as asbestosis. There is a treatment, but there is no cure. He was diagnosed as having asbestosis in April 1968 and told he had less than five years to live. Six months prior to that, after completing the regular series of x-rays and full physical with the J-M plant physician, he had been pronounced fit.[1]

In the spring of 1977 parents of young children in the United States were advised that the bulk of the sleepwear that they had purchased for their children contained a chemical, Tris, that might condemn a proportion—small, but nonetheless significant—of those children to death or disability from cancer some twenty years from now. Tris, a chemical developed as a flame retardant with the best of motives, also turns out to be one of the most potent carcinogens. For those children already exposed to Tris the damage is irreversible.

In June 1973 a toxic flame retardant called Firemaster was accidentally mixed into livestock feed distributed by the Farm Bureau Services, an affiliate of Michigan's agricultural trade association. More than 30,000 cattle, 2 million chickens, and thousands of sheep and hogs who ate the feed either died soon thereafter or became so sick they had to be prematurely slaughtered by farmers. The chemical that caused all the problems, commonly called PBB, created an irrversible chemical contamination not only of the animals exposed to it but of those human being subsequently exposed to the chemical through ingestion of contaminated meat products. In 1976 the Michigan Department of Public Health revealed that about 96 percent of the nursing mothers tested had PBB in their milk and in many cases well beyond the level of contamination allowed in cow's milk.

There are a number of ways to look at the subject of corporate responsibility for health. The assumption of responsibility by employers for the medical care benefits of their employees is a relatively recent phenomenon. Corporations have long assumed some responsibility for the health and safety of their workers on the job, and to a lesser degree for the quality of the environment in which they do business. And all are health-related responsibilities. Inevitably the first receives the greatest attention. Yet corporate responsibility for environmental quality may hold far greater health payoffs, not only to the company and its employees, but to society as well.

The Role of the Corporation: Medical Care or Health?

As evidence mounts that modern medical care is reaching the limits of its capacity to contribute to the health of the population in the United States, the relative importance of the other determinants of health increased. What that may mean is that the corporate role in job safety and environmental quality may be more productive than its role as the guarantor of employee medical care benefits.

The history of medicine is characterized by the progressive specialization of medical technique. Medicine began essentially as a social science; it had few if any effective technologies. Then, as it benefited from the scientific revolution of the nineteenth century, it slowly incorporated some scientific principles and methods, principally those that aided it in detecting the specific agents of disease. This resulted, among other things, in the schism between public health focused on population measures, and medical care which translated the emerging scientific understanding of disease into specific treatment programs for individual patients.

The diagnosis and treatment of individuals has continued to be the emphasis of medicine since early in this century. Medicine is far from a mature science, but it is an evolving one. This evolution has been fueled by a steady flow of information about human biology. Patients today benefit from an impressive body of knowledge and technique. Yet as it has evolved, medicine has necessarily emphasized some of the variables related to health and disease to the relative neglect of others. Because of the emphasis in research on the biochemical nature of disease, those variables associated with biochemical processes are better understood than those associated with behavior, sociocultural factors, and environment variables. And existing research agendas promise an even further unfolding of the biochemical nature of disease. Given these agendas, the issue is whether the knowledge already gained, together with the knowledge to be gained from further research, is sufficient to equip the medical care practitioner with the tools he or she needs to control today's major health problems.

What is the likelihood of breakthroughs in basic research focused on today's major health problems similar to those of the past that enabled medicine to control many of the major infectious diseases? This question cannot be answered definitively. There are many who believe that such breakthroughs are just around the corner. Others are less optimistic, and still others doubt that such breakthroughs are likely, either because the costs of their achievement are too high, or because today's major diseases are unlikely to be amenable to the sort of technology that can be produced by current research approaches. Those who argue the latter case often contend that today's major diseases are more likely to be controlled through a more precise understanding of the relationship of behavioral, sociocultural, and environmental variables.

What does this mean to today's corporation?

What is the Corporation's Reponsibility?

In 1962 the University of Pittsburgh in a massive study investigated the relationship between the causes of death among steelworkers and their work histories. A pattern soon became evident. Cancer of the lung, bronchus, and trachea was killing white steelworkers at a rate 28 percent greater than whites in the general population. For nonwhite workers—those generally stuck with the worst jobs—the rate was 64 percent greater than nonwhites in general population. In other words, the expected fatality rate for these sorts of cancers—3 for every 100 deaths—became nearly 8 out of 100 for workers in the steel industry.

Larry Agran, in his book *The Cancer Connection*, includes a number of similar examples. Rubber workers develop cancers at a rate of 50 percent to 300 percent greater than the general population. Coke oven workers die of lung cancer five to six times more frequently than the general population. Asbestos workers, even those with short-term exposures, die of lung cancer at a rate more than seven times that of control groups. Nearly all of a group of dyestuff workers—94 percent—developed bladder tumors after five years or more of occupational exposure. Miners also succumb to many occupationally induced cancers; among uranium miners, for instance, over 50 percent of all deaths are due to lung cancer. Perhaps 2 million workers in a wide variety of industries are exposed to the solvent benzine, a known cause of leukemia. Another 1.5 million laborers are exposed to the carcinogen inorganic arsenic. And the list of special cancer risks could go on and on.[2]

As Agran points out, this epidemic has just recently emerged, since in many cases the exposure to chemicals does not manifest in disease until many years later. Even more recently, the General Accounting Office estimated that American workers may be exposed to as many as 1,500 substances that could cause cancer. Unfortunately, the government has established safety standards for only 15 of them. The GAO in its report stated that the bleak occupational health conditions that Congress tried to improve by passing the OSHAct still exist and may be getting worse. The report estimates that each year 390,000 new cases of occupational diesease appear. Yet at the rate the government is issuing standards on toxic substances and work environments, the goal of protecting workers from these hazards will not be achieved at any time soon.

The point is simple. We may be on the verge of an epidemic of occupational disease, much of it cancer, and still most of it undiscovered. Yet daily, new chemicals are introduced into the workplace and chemicals already in use continue to be used despite many well-founded suspicions that they may be disease-producing and in many cases carcinogenic. The government, principally through OSHA, has offered a feeble response. Again, as in many other cases, the question then ultimately becomes one of corporate responsiblity. There is no doubt, upon examination of some of the above case histories and in the investigative work done to build those cases, that industry has not only been lax in the enforcement of established standards, it has been singularly unwilling to test or to offer for testing chemicals that it proposes to use in the course of doing business.

If the GAO estimate is accurate, nearly 100,000 persons will die in the United States this year and in each ensuing year as a result of occupationally induced disease. What are the comparable health-related impacts of the provision of employee medical care benefits? Is it likely that lavish corporate attention to the provision of employee medical benefits could reduce human loss by as many as 100,000 lives per year?

There is a related issue. It is one thing to argue that corporations possess the responsibility for improving the quality of the workplace, but it is another to say that corporations possess the responsibility to improve the quality of the environment at large. Yet through the manufacture and distribution of chemicals like Tris and PBB, untold morbidity and mortality results. There is no suggestion here (nor for that matter in most of the literature on this subject), that the introduction of those chemicals by the companies responsible was willful and malicious. At worst it might be said that those companies might have been aware of the potential disease-producing nature of those chemicals but chose to remain silent. Yet this is heinous enough. But take the PBB example a little further. The discovery of the harmful nature of the chemical should properly lead to a ban on its further use. But the point is that the introduction of the chemical in the first place caused irreversible effects in the life-chain itself. Not only were cattle and other animals harmed, but many humans, including suckling infants and breast-feeding mothers, clearly were also harmed. And because of the potency and "durability" of the chemical, it will remain in the life-chain for many more years.

Again, the tragedy is that since the results of the activity of the chemical are so delayed, we really will not know the true impact on human health for another twenty years or so. This is the case with a number of other chemicals as well. The question is: Is industry willing to voluntarily assume more responsibility not only to its workers but to all the rest of us, not only for damage done, but for damage being done and damage about to be done through the indiscriminate development, distribution, and use of chemicals with either known or suspected disease-producing properties?

NOTES

1. *Newsleads*, vol. 6 (Los Angeles: Urban Policy Research Institute, February-March 1977).

2. Larry Agran, *The Cancer Connection* (New York: Houghton Mifflin, 1977).

Growing Legal Liability in Corporate Health Clinics

John D. Blum

17

Dramatic· escalation of health care costs has led industry to explore alternatives to the traditional medical insurance coverage in constructing employee benefit packages. The desire to limit costs has spawned a movement toward the expansion of in-house clinics to provide more comprehensive services beyond their traditional diagnostic and testing services, first aid, and emergency treatment. However, a number of issues must be resolved prior to a significant corporate commitment in this area. A major concern is the question corporate liability implications of enlarging the tasks of company clinics, specifically, whether a corporation can be held liable for the negligent conduct of a physician providing medical treatment in a company clinic.

The Employer's Duty to Provide Health Services

Historically, an employer had no duty under the common law to provide medical services for his employees.[1] However, in a number of cases involving railroad accidents, various state courts have held that in an emergency accident situation, an employer does have a responsibility to see that medical assistance is provided. Over time there has developed a general duty for the employer to provide assistance if an employee has sustained a serious, life-threatening injury on the job. In the case of *Batton v. Atlantic Coast Line Railroad Co.* the court stated that, "there is a tendency . . . to hold that where in the course of his employment a servant suffers serious injury or is suddenly stricken down in a manner indicating immediate and emergent need of aid to save him from death or serious harm, the master, if present, is bound to take such reasonable measure or make such reasonable effort as may be practical to relieve him, even though the master is not chargeable with fault in bringing about the emergency."[2] The employer's duty to assist after an accident it is not, however, an absolute responsibility. It is contingent on the extent of the injury, in some cases on the kind of industry, and on whether corporate negligence was involved.

In situations where an employee becomes ill at work, the duty under the common law to assist is not as clear as in an accident situation. The extent of the corporation's responsibility in this case depends upon how visibly ill the worker appears and upon the accessibility of medical services; aiding employees who are taken ill is often a moral rather than a legal responsibility. However, once the employer comes to the assistance of the employee, that assistance must be provided with appropriate care as required under the general principles of tort law.[3]

A factor in the increasing availability of on-site health services is the Occupational Safety and Health Act (OSHAct) of 1970.[4] While OSHAct has been subject to widespread criticism and even labeled a bureaucractic boondoggle, it has been responsible for an increased awareness on the part of both labor and management of the need to combat health hazards.* OSHAct requires that workers exposed to certain toxic materials or high levels of radiation receive periodic physical examinations and diagnostic screening, and that industries provide medical treatment on the premises or have it readily available in the immediate vicinity.[5] OSHAct's basic thrust is toward creating a safe work environment through area safety standards rather than through requiring specific kinds of medical facilities on the premises. The administering agency has, however, recently upgraded its screening requirements for corporations utilizing toxic substances; such regulatory activity will force expansion of in-house clinics in certain industries.[6]

Dramatic findings of widespread worker exposure to carcinogens has joined legislative activity in heightening public awareness of occupational hazards.[7] Episodes involving black lung disease, asbestos, kepone, PCB, and vinyl chloride poisoning have created a conviction that in situations where corporations expose their employees to a health risk, those corporations must combat that risk or face potential corporate liability.

Another source of the corporate duty to provide medical services is the

*The recently passed Toxic Substance Control Act (Pub. L. 94-469) is intended to fill OSHAct's gaps in the area of chemical substances and mixtures. This act is designed to avoid potential harm new chemicals may cause by requiring that anyone exposed to a risk be adequately notified.

employment contract. Generally, employee contracts (union or not) do not delineate the specific kinds of medical services to be provided, but indicate only the overall health plans agreed upon.* There are, however, circumstances under which a contractual obligation will be found, or alternatively, under which corporate liability will arise from breach of contract.

Corporate Liability under Workmen's Compensation Laws

Almost all injuries that occur at the workplace are compensable under the state no-fault Workmen's Compensation (WC) system. In recent years the coverage of WC laws has been expanded well beyond the on-the-job accident situation; there are now only a handful of states that still limit compensation to accidents arising out of, or in the course of, employment.[8] Compensation is now afforded for aggravation or acceleration of a preexisting weakness; the theory is that an employer hires a worker with the risk that a prior condition could be aggravated on the job. WC did not originally cover diseases, but gradually there developed a judicial recognition that physical ailments that grow over time as a result of exposure to dangerous pollutants constitute a work injury. The move to reimburse workers for diseases incurred on the job was sparked by findings of serious, life-threatening illness developed by employees in certain industries.[9] Initially, states created listings of diseases included under compensation statues; presently, many jurisdictions cover under WC laws all diseases that are work-related.**

The scope of WC laws has been broadened by courts to a point perhaps well beyond the intent of the lawmakers. For example, injuries occurring during lunch hour athletic pursuits are now regularly held compensable.[10] Still, no matter how broad the extension of benefits made by the WC panel or state courts, there must always be a showing that a causal connection exists between the physical infirmity and the employment involved. Problems arise concerning the causal connection in such cases as stress and tension injuries, especially heart attacks.†

---

*In some cases union health and welfare trust fund administrators have the power to determine the kinds of health services members will be entitled to.

**One should note that WC laws vary from state to state. It is difficult to generalize about their application but it is still safe to argue that in all jurisdictions their scope has been significantly broadened.

†The court in the New Jersey case of *Walck v. Johns-Manville Products Co.* stated the general rule that "heart attacks to be compensable must arise out of employment and be due in some realistic and material degree to risk reasonably incident to employment; it must issue from or be contributed to by conditions which bear some essential relation to work or its nature." A California court of appeals in *Kaiser-Permanente v. Worker's Compensation Appeal Board* held that a presumption of occupational disease would be applied in the case of a policeman who suffered a heart attack a year after retirement when there was documented evidence to verify that he had suffered from heart trouble during employment. No state, however liberal its WC laws, will award compensation in cases where a causal link cannot be demonstrated between the injury in question and the nature of the employment.

In considering WC laws in relation to medical malpractice, the initial question is whether an employee who has sustained a work-related injury can collect under WC for aggravation of that injury through malpractice. WC awards will generally cover medical expenses for negligently aggravated injuries. In *Manly v. American Packing Co.* the court stated that "it is a well recognized principle of WC law that injuries which follow as legitimate consequences of the original accident are compensable and such accident need not have been the sole or direct cause of the condition complained of."[11] In other words, one can recover under WC for injuries that stem directly from physician negligence even if they are not related to the initial injury for which the employee is visiting the clinic.* For purposes of compensation it does not matter whether the negligent physician was an employee of the corporation or was the worker's private physician. In order for an award to be made, it must be demonstrated that there exists no intervening independent cause to break the chain of negligence between the aggravated and the original injury.

In a majority of jurisdictions the injured worker has the right to bring suit for malpractice against the physician who treated the work-related injury. The right to sue a negligent physician is allowed in some jurisdictions even after a worker has received WC benefits that reimburse for the negligently induced injury. In the North Carolina case of *Bryant v. Dougherty* the court ruled that the WC laws do not affect nor should recovery under them prejudice the right of the injured worker to maintain a separate negligence action against the treating physician.[12] An Iowa court in *Bradshaw v. Iowa Methodist Hospital* stated, "[O]ur compensation law does not abolish common law actions in tort except those between employer and employee. The provision in the act that the rights provided for an employee on account of an injury shall be exclusive of all other rights of such employees applies only to actions against the employer, and does not prevent an injured employee from suing third persons at common law."[13] The rationale for allowing recovery both under WC and in tort is that the former system is a no-fault arrangement between employer and employee; a physician as a third party is not privy to that relationship and thus generally falls outside the scope of the state WC acts.

Some state laws allow a worker to maintain a separate action against a negligent physician provided that the worker was not awarded special damages under WC for the injuries resulting from malpractice. Thus, two separate suits can be maintained only if the WC award is limited to compensation for the initial injury (generally these laws require some type of election of remedy). A Maine court in *Steeves v. Irwin* stated that, generally, a separate lawsuit could be maintained for negligence against a physician unless the amount paid on the judgment or in consideration of the release constitutes full compensation for the employee's injuries inflicted both by the original tortfeasor and by the negligent physician.[14] In Massachusetts the law allows an employee the option to proceed either against the negligent third-party physician or the compensa-

---

*This does not mean that when an employee visits a clinic for a non-work-related injury or illness that WC will cover.

tion insurer; in addition, the insurer can bring suit within nine months against a third party for damages paid out to the employee, but if the insurer fails to exercise the right it passes back to the employee. The court in *Turner v. Guiliano* stated that under Massachusetts law, even if the right to sue the third-party physician passed back, if the employee had already recovered the doctrine of unjust enrichment would preclude a second action.[15]

Subrogation of the right to sue is often required where an employee's claim has been satisfied through WC. In *Overbeek v. Nex* a Michigan court took the position that where an employee had collected in full for an injury under compensation provisions, the right to sue the negligent physician passed by subrogation to the employer.[16] In *Pitkin v. Chapman* a New York court stated that "there can be but one recovery for the same wrong; . . . satisfaction by one joint tortfeasor has always been considered a bar to an action against another . . . the WC act provided that where another party or wholly responsible for the injury, the one paying shall be subrogated to the remedy of the employee against the other."[17] In some states the failure of a party to exercise subrogation rights allows the employee to pursue the action. In the state of Maine, for instance, if the employee recovers he may sue the third party if the subrogated right is not enforced, thus taking advantage of a double recovery. In *Steeves v. Irwin* the court recognized that the right to sue the treating physician passed back to the employee at the WC hearing when both the employer and the insurer made it clear they did not intend to pursue the matter.[18]

In a number of jurisdictions WC laws contain the fellow-servant doctrine—immunity provisions that preclude one employee from suing another for a work-related injury. The crucial issue regarding company medical malpractice is whether the physician is considered a fellow worker. Many courts do not view the physician as an employee or agent of the corporation within the scope of the WC laws and thus have not applied this provision (see below). In the case of *Proctor v. Ford Motor Co.*, however, an Ohio court ruled that a full-time, salaried physician is protected under the immunity provisions of the WC laws. The court pointed out that in order for Ohio's immunity statute not to apply to company physicians, their employment must be both casual and not in the ordinary course of business.[19] In instances where an immunity rule precludes suit against a fellow-employee physician (such instances are now the exception), WC would be the exclusive remedy for incidents of medical negligence that arise in this context.

A related issue is whether double recovery is permitted where an employee is covered under a personal accident, hospital, or medical insurance policy. Generally, most health insurance policies specify that in the event the insured recovers under WC for an injury, additional compensation will not be forthcoming (even if the employee agrees to turn over insurance proceeds to the employer). Some policies contain clauses that reduce the liability of the insurer depending upon the size of the award under WC. In cases where an insurance policy does not address this issue (which is rare), the rule is established that recovery under WC does not preclude compensation under the policy.[20]

Corporate Liability Other Than Workmen's Compensation

Workmen's Compensation acts as a buffer to corporate liability for physician negligence whenever a causal connection can be established between work setting and injury. It is only where there is no such connection that the issue of corporate liability for malpractice becomes significant. If an employee is treated in a company clinic for a non-work-related condition, and is subsequently injured through the treatment, state WC laws would not apply. It is, however, not always easy to draw the line between work-related and non-work-related injury. In the New York case of *Garcia v. Iseron* the plaintiff was injured by an improperly administered injection in the company clinic. While the injection probably could not be seen as work-related, the New York court viewed it as being a unique service that was a consequence of employment, thus falling under WC recovery.[21] This ruling, while illustrative of the difficulties in distinguishing work-related injuries, should not be interpreted too broadly, since it dealt with a service that was given as a matter of routine to all employees. The malpractice situations that may lead to corporate liability outside WC are those where special services are improperly administered to an employee on a selective basis.

There are two principles on which the liability of a corporation for the malpractice of a company physician may be based: the responsibility of a corporation to employ competent physicians, and the doctrine of respondeat superior from which one can develop a corporate benefits theory and an independent contractual argument.

A corporation that supplies medical treatment to its workers has a clear duty to exercise reasonable care in ensuring that the practitioners it employes are competent. In a rare situation where a company hires (or contracts with) a practitioner who it knows or should have known was not qualified, corporate liability will arise. The case law in this area often distinguishes between situations where the employer supplies medical treatment gratuitously and those where care is provided under a statutory or contractual obligation. Where health care is given gratuitously, the traditional rule has been that the employer's only liability stems from the failure to hire qualified medical personnel.[22] In *Chicago B & O Railroad Co. v. Howard* the court stated the general rule, "the employer was only required to select persons possessing the degree of knowledge and skill ordinarily possessed by members of the medical profession, and was not responsible for the physicians employed by it . . .[I]t would be absurd to insist not only that the selection should be prudent, but that the company should guarantee that the physicians selected would make no mistakes and be guilty of no negligence."[23] In a later case involving the liability of a railroad physician, a North Carolina court reiterated this rule of law, "the only duty which the employer owes the employee is to exercise reasonable care in the selection and employment of the physician . . . [T]he employer will not be held liable for damages resulting from the unskilled or negligent treatment of the employee."[24] The number of cases where a corporation has actually been found liable for gratuitously providing medical services through employment of an incompetent physician is quite small, especially in recent years.[25]

Few actions have been brought addressing the question whether the corporation has a broader liability if it is obligated to provide health services beyond the well-recognized responsibility for hiring competent physicians. A number of older cases in Texas and Washington take the position that if an employer has a contractual obligation to supply employees with health care, the scope of liability is extended.[26] A California appellate court in *Bowman v. Southern Pacific Co.* ruled that an employer who is supplying substantial medical services funded by employee wage deductions, incurs a corporate liability for the negligent conduct of physicians it employs.[27] The nature of the employment contract in question will have bearing upon how far a court is able to extend the scope of corporate responsibility.

On the other hand, there is authority that holds that for liability purposes it does not matter why the health services are provided. In *Smith v. Buckeye Cotton Oil Co.* the court ruled that whether the employer owes an employee the duty of furnishing medical care or it is done gratuitously, the only possible liability stems from lack of due care in selection.[28] Courts have viewed the provision of medical services beyond the scope of a specific duty as being something done for the employees' benefit without profit or gain to the employer, and the corporation is thus subjected to only minimal liability for physician error. Other courts have protected corporations from liability when providing health care services on the theory of charitable immunity.[29]

The duty of the corporation to hire competent medical personnel includes a responsibility not to retain the services of a physician who becomes unfit over time. Indeed, this expansion of corporate responsibility is a logical out-growth of the duty to utilize skilled physicians; in *Ashby v. Davis Coal and Coke Co.* the court expressed the duty of a corporation to hire and retain a competent physician as being one and the same responsibility.[30]

This duty requires some kind of monitoring of physician behavior. The role of the corporation as a monitor of its medical services may in fact be significantly extended with an increase in corporate clinic services. The company that provides employee medical services directly is producing health care as one of its products; it in fact takes on a role analogous to other health care institutions. Under the current law of some states, hospitals have an affirmative duty both to monitor their medical care and to ensure that an acceptable level of quality is maintained.* The expansion of the hospital's duty in the quality monitoring area in the well-known case of *Darling v. Charlestown Community Hospital* has grown to where hospitals are required to develop functioning quality assurance programs.[31]

If the expanded corporate clinic is viewed as another kind of provider institution, one may by analogy argue that the corporation has an affirmative duty to monitor the quality of care delivered in its clinics, and that the failure to do so adequately may entail liability. Under this theory, a peer review program

---

*Such a responsibility arises also from the Joint Commission on Accreditation of Hospitals program and from obligations under Medicare and Medicaid.

may have to be established that is more than a claims review mechanism.[32] The likelihood of applying a quality assurance responsibility to a corporation will depend on how extensive are the services it provides in-house, and in the long range on what kind of tie-in industry will have with national health insurance.*

The doctrine of respondeat superior, often referred to as the master-servant doctrine or in its broadest sense as vicarious liability, holds that an employer is liable for the tortious conduct of his employees or agent.** Respondeat superior does not apply where an employer enters into a relationship with an independent contractor. Traditionally, many courts have viewed the status of a hired company physician as that of an independent contractor, thus precluding employer liability for the physician's negligence. The court in the Kentucky case of *Western Union Telegraph Co. v. Mason* stated that the widely held rule that "the employer cannot direct the physician as to the mode of treatment and has no control over him, except the right to discharge him . . . and thus the rule of respondeat superior did not apply."[33] In *Schneider v. New York Telephone Co.* it was reasoned that even though the physician in question was regularly employed by the company, he was engaged in an independent calling and thus his status was deemed to be an independent contractor.[34] The primary concern in assessing whether respondeat superior should apply is the degree of control exercised by the employer over the actions of the employee. In the case of the company physician, corporations have generally exercised only a power of dismissal; they exert very little control over physician practices.

The doctrine of respondeat superior should not, however, be dismissed, for in some instances it may be used to establish employer liability. Many of the cases that ruled out vicarious liability in the employer-physician relationship were litigated well before the expanded provision of employee health services. The current trend in the law is shifting toward an expansion of respondeat superior to include professional employees and agents.[35]

The initial expansion of vicarious liability occurred in situations where corporations exercised a higher degree of control over physician behavior than usual. A federal court in *O'Donnell v. Pennsylvania Railroad Co.* held that "where a company physician took general orders from superiors who could make recommendations or suggestions about medical treatment and the physician had a social security number, a service record, a wage record and worked regular hours . . . the physician under such circumstances was an employee of the company whose negligence the company was responsible for."[36] Another federal court applying Mississippi law in *Knox v. Ingalls Shipbuilding Co.* stated that "the principal is responsible for the tort of his agent, not because the former has done wrong, but because the law so declares as a matter of public policy and there is not more reason to except employers of physicians from the

*In a national health insurance plan requiring employer contributions, companies may offer extensive in-house health services as an option to their workers in hopes of reducing company costs. Such decisions may lead to mandated peer reviews in these company clinics.

**Application of the master-servant doctrine does not prevent the injured party from suing both the tortfeasor and the employer separately.

doctrine of respondeat superior than there is to exempt employers of other highly skilled persons who perform technical services requiring discretion."[37] In a recent California case the court treated physicians who were employed full-time like any other kind of employee for negligence purposes.[38]

The respondeat superior doctrine is significantly strengthened by the existence of a contractual duty to provide the services for which the employer-physician relationship is undertaken. In such a situation the physician becomes a corporate agent carrying out its duty. There are two theories of contract law that can be utilized to demonstrate that the provision of health care provided by a corporation is pursuant to a contractual obligation: the doctrine of promissory estoppel and the third-party beneficiary contract.

Whether a corporation has an express contractual obligation to provide in-house health services will depend upon the terms of the employment contract. In some instances employee contracts may be quite specific concerning the kinds of health benefits to be provided. This is rare, however, and it can be difficult to determine whether the provision of medical services in a company clinic is a contractual right. Corporations are likely to see clinics as fringe benefits created at the discretion of the company as a gratuitous incident to employment—even when employees indirectly contribute to funding those clinics. Only those screening procedures required under OSHAct for certain industries would definitely be considered a corporate duty and this responsibility does not stem from employment contracts.

The argument could be made, however, that under the rules of contract law where a corporate health clinic is in existence at the time an employee is hired, its presence could be reasonably relied upon by the employee. Continued existence of the health facility constitutes a contractual obligation if it is likely thata worker would come to expect medical services to be provided there. The contractual doctrine invoked here is that of promissory estoppel, which holds that "a promise which the promisor should reasonably expect to induce action or forbearance on the part of the promisee which does induce such action or forbearance is binding."[39] The promissory estoppel doctrine has been broadly liberalized and expanded from a gift-giving situation to use in a commercial setting.[40]

Certainly, it is reasonable for an employee to rely upon in-house health services as an incident of employment, and thus it could be argued that an employer's attempt to withdraw such services might be construed as a breach of contract.* Whether promissory estoppel can further serve to uphold a legal responsibility to provide specific kinds of services in-house depends upon the representation made to the employees and on a determination of whether it was reasonable for the employee to feel that the specific services in question were an incident of employment.

A more tenable argument can be made using the doctrine of the third-party beneficiary contract to demonstrate a legal obligation to provide in-house

---

*An express promise to offer in-house health services is not necessary, indications to the employee that such medical services are available may be sufficient to justify reliance and support a promissory estoppel argument.

health services to employees. The third-party beneficiary contract arises where an agreement is entered into between two parties for the benefit of a third.[41] In order for the doctrine to apply, the benefit in question must run directly to the third party and be designed primarily for that individual. It does not matter whether the third party has a right to receive the benefits; even if the benefits are conferred as a gratuity, the third party can enforce the contract between the initial parties. In the employee health situation the worker can be viewed as a third-party beneficiary of the agreement between the corporation and the company physician to provide services in the company clinic. There is no question that the employer-physician agreement is designed for the direct benefit of the employee (even though it is often more beneficial to the employer, see below), and respondeat superior therefore applies.

The third-party beneficiary contract may have even broader ramifications. A worker may be able to directly sue a corporation for damages caused by the malpractice of a company physician on the grounds that the contractual agreement entered into for his benefit was violated. Negligent conduct in pursuance of a contractual obligation can be, if it is serious enough, grounds for breach of contract. In the agreement made between physician and corporation to provide medical services, as in all contracts, there is an implied condition that the physician will render treatment pursuant to the agreement in a nonnegligent fashion.[42] Failure to honor the contract, by delivering substandard medical care or performing negligently, violates a contractual condition of performance and can lead to a damage suit by the third-party beneficiary, the employee.*

One might argue that the corporation has no duty to supply in-house health services to its employees, but enters into a contract with a physician to provide such services only as a gratuity. There is thus no obligation running between company and employee on which to base the third-party beneficiary contract theory. While a corporation may not have an express obligation to deliver medical services in a corporate clinic, once it contracts with someone to provide such services, even as a gratuity, there exists a responsibility to honor that obligation. While the employee may not be a creditor beneficiary (one whom the employer owes an obligation), he is a donee beneficiary of the physician-employer agreement, and this position creates a legal right of enforcement.

Another derivative theory based on the respondeat superior or vicarious liability doctrine that can be used to demonstrate corporate liability for in-house physician negligence is the company benefits argument. Basically, if a corporation establishes in-house clinics for its own advantage or purposes, the physicians who assist the company in achieving those goals are acting as

*In some instances where a company physician refuses to provide services agreed upon in the physician-employer contract, the employee may sue for restoration of services or for monetary compensation as a result of having to seek outside medical assistance. In a third-party beneficiary situation, the third party can bring suit against either of the initial contracting parties and those parties in turn may have rights against each another. The cause of action by the employee beneficiary lies in contract and so it is not the negligent act itself that is the focal point of the action, but the fact the contracting parties failed to live up to their obligation to the third party.

agents of the corporation, and thus the company is liable for physician misconduct under respondeat superior.

The company benefits argument can be traced to a situation where a
corporation actually received a financial profit by establishing its own health
plan. In the 1899 case of *Texas and Pacific Coal Co. v. Connaughton* the
company collected a compulsory wage deduction for physician services that
resulted in a substantial surplus in its bank account. The Texas court held that
such a health plan was for employer profit and thus the company was liable for
the resultant malpractice.[43] In a similar case a Pennsylvania court reasoned that
the company that gains from providing health services should be treated for
liability purposes as though it were a medical provider.[44]

With changes in employee health packages and escalating costs, the
return a corporation can derive from creating in-house health plans has
changed from a profit to a stimulant for cost savings in health benefits area.
Courts have labeled the cost-saving capability of a health plan as a benefit upon
which liability can be incurred when physicians acting to effect company
health goals are negligent. In the California case of *McGuigan v. Southern
Pacific Co.* the court stated that in the employee health area, "the key test as to
the extent of the employer's duty is whether the employer secures a financial
benefit in the operation of the health facility, if so, the employer is liable for the
negligence of the physicians performing a duty assumed by the employer."[45] In
the case of *Mangrum v. Union Pacific Co.* the court attached liability to the
corporation for physician negligence on "the theory that the physician was
engaged in an operational activity of the defendant railroad necessary in
carrying out its franchise, since the railroad can't operate with a healthy crew,
and on the theory that a financial benefit accrued to the railroad from the
doctor's service since it was required by custom and practice to take care of its
employees who were sick on duty."[46] In *Knox v. Ingalls* a Mississippi court
concluded that the company clinic (which injured employees were required to
use) was established for corporate purposes, and thus the physicians working
in the clinic were agents for whose actions the company was responsible.[47]

The case law supporting the benefits argument is fairly conclusive that
respondeat superior will apply where evidence demonstrates that the corporate
health plan is created for company benefit.* The difficulty with this theory is in
determining when a health facility functions primarily for the benefit of the
corporation. Clearly, whatever health services the company provides are of
benefit to the worker who receives treatment, but this fact does not detract from
the argument that the clinic or medical service was established primarily for
the company's benefit. This benefit theory is especially applicable to the on-site
company facility because the chances are good that there will be savings to the
corporation resulting from decreased worker time loss and increase operational
efficiency. The Ohio Supreme Court in the case of *Proctor v. Ford Motor Co.*
made an interesting observation about the corporate benefits of an in-house
health care facility: "The business of Ford is manufacturing automobiles; yet to

---

*The cases cited in this section involved situations where the employee made significant
contributions to the health plan. As the law is currently developing, the benefit theory is not
influenced by this fact because even where the employer pays most of the cost, a significant corporate
benefit may still be realized.

say that its maintenance of a full staffed plant medical facility is unrelated to producing cars ignores the reality of modern industrial life. Ford's business interest in efficiency of operation is directly served by providing readily accessible medical care to those workmen whose minor injuries or ailments might otherwise result in their absence from the production line . . . So while there is no doubt that the workmen are most directly served by a plant dispensary, it is equally clear that appellant physicians are employed in work that furthers the business interests of their employer."[48]

Where the services provided by the corporation in-house are more comprehensive, the question of benefits to the corporation will be more difficult to determine. There may be situations where some types of medical services delivered will not result in cost or time savings or other recognized corporate advantages, and could be provided more cheaply through outside alternatives; here the benefits argument may not be applicable. While some courts have viewed benefits in terms of savings and efficiency, the problem is complicated because others have used the term very generally, failing to specify what exactly the benefit in question entailed. Thus, even when a corporation's clinic does not produce savings, a court may construe other types of benefits (for instance, worker satisfaction) on which to base a vicarious liability argument.

A question that warrants separate attention is whether a corporation can be held liable for events arising out of employment physical examinations and other medical screening programs. In this situation, two possible situations can entail employer liability: failure to inform workers about adverse medical conditions and lack of due care in conducting the examination or screening procedure.[49]

The employer is generally under no duty to provide physical examinations (with the exception of OSHA requirements in certain industries). However, once he undertakes to perform a physical examination, there is authority to the effect that responsibility exists to inform the worker of any adverse findings.[50] In the California case of *Vela v. Wise* a lower court ruled that a company physician employed by Johns-Manville failed to live up to a duty to inform a worker that he had contracted asbestosis, and was thus personally liable (the company in turn could be held liable under the respondeat superior argument).[51] It is necessary, of course, in cases dealing with the corporation's failure to inform employees about adverse medical conditions that proof be presented showing that the employer had actual or presumed knowledge about the workers' physical conditions; without such a showing liability will not attach.*

A related issue is whether failure to inform a worker about an adverse medical condition (or misdiagnosis of a condition) would be compensable under Workmen's Compensation laws. In the Texas case of *Lotspeich v. Chance Vought Aircraft* the court held that the WC law was the exclusive remedy between employee and employer where there was alleged injury through failure to inform about an adverse medical finding.[52] The Texas court

---

*Certain types of medical reports are filed routinely by company physicians with their employers. For a discussion of corporate medical files and confidentiality, see George J. Annas, "Legal Aspects of Medical Confidentiality in the Occupational Setting," *Journal of Occupational Medicine,* vol. 18, no. 8, August 1976.

was of the opinion (as most courts would be) that an individual in a preemployment physical examination is an employee for purposes of compensation because the examination is conducted exclusively for the employer's benefit. A New York court faced with the same issue in *Wojeik v. Aluminum Co.* took the position that the state WC law was not the sole remedy for a worker injured through failure to inform, but an independent cause of action could be sustained.[53] Whether WC laws will be an exclusive remedy in this kind of situation is thus a matter of how state courts interpret these laws.[54]

There is no duty on the part of an employer to discover an employee's illness; courts that have framed the corporate responsibility in such a light (as in *Lotspeich*) have misinterpreted the issue. The corporation has a duty to ensure that due care is exercised by their physician agents in performing examinations or diagnostic screening procedures. Failure to discover an adverse physical condition or misdiagnosis should lead only to vicarious liability for the employer where a company physician failed to exercise due care.

The extent of the corporation's liability for company physician misdiagnosis depends upon the purpose for which the examination or screening process is conducted. If the examination is performed to determined fitness for a given task and the negligent failure to detect some adverse condition will jeopardize a worker's health, then clearly corporate liability should arise from such an oversight. In *Coffee v. McDonnell Douglas* the employer's failure to take into account the result of a blood test that demonstrated a direct risk to an employee pilot was clearly negligent; the duty of an employer dealing with another kind of employee may not be deemed that extensive.[55]

Another basis of liability derives from faulty operating procedures in an employee clinic. In *McGuigan v. Southern Pacific Co.* the corporation was held to be independently negligent because it improperly assigned work responsibilities to an individual who it should have known was not physically capable of such an assignment. The corporation had failed to take into consideration information it possessed as a result of physical examinations (in this case there was no process for sharing adverse medical information with either the employee or management).[56] In *Coffee* the company was held to be independently liable for the failure to establish adequate procedures for the evaluation of blood test reports.[57] What *McGuigan*, *Coffee*, and similar cases seem to be leading to is a doctrine of corporate liability arising from the overall failure to establish an adequate in-house clinic, a doctrine going beyond vicarious liability for physician negligence or the failure to hire competent medical personnel and monitor medical staff behavior.

Minimizing the Risk of Malpractice Liability in Corporate Clinics

Corporate liability for physician misconduct is not yet a major problem, but it is a key factor in decisions about expanding in-house medical facilities. This presentation of the bases for corporate liability is not meant to paint expansion as an ill-advised step; where cost savings can be realized the advantages may outweigh the risks. The corporation must, however, recognize that the expansion of services increases risk exposure and may in fact create new liabilities. In approaching the question of how to combat potential liability for physician negligence, corporations should consider the following:

The scope of coverage for in-house malpractice incidents provided under that state's Workmen's Compensation laws. In some states WC coverage may be broad enough to include such injuries.

The possibility of increasing liability insurance coverage. Some corporations have self-insured for WC; this approach may be feasible to cover potential corporate malpractice claims.

Developing a well-defined policy of what services to perform in the clinic. Outside of an emergency situation, no services other than those specifically agreed upon should be provided. Employees should be made aware of what services are available and a referral mechanism should be created for treatment that is not available in-house.

Instituting a form of in-house quality assurance (peer review, medical audit) to ensure a high level of treatment. It would also be desirable for corporate clinics to undergo some kind of outside evaluation on a regular basis.

A system for reporting suspected malpractice problems to the company medical director, and if appropriate, to the company legal counsel. If the medical staff conduct epidemiological studies on the worker population that uncover negative results, such results should be passed on to management and, if significant enough, to the employees.

Worker access to their own medical records. If a physical examination uncovers a condition that negatively affects job performance, the company physician has a duty to so inform the worker. In serious conditions of physical impairment, the corporation should be informed. This presents a serious problem in that such information should not be used to force a worker off the job. It is often in fact so used. Medical information that does not deal directly with the ability of a worker to perform on the job should be held in confidence between physician and employee.

Finally, it is worth stating the obvious: corporate negligence for medical malpractice will only be a problem where company physicians fail to exercise due care or obtain informed consent. It is thus important that companies hire competent practitioners, provide them with adequate facilities and support personnel, and assign them realistic case loads. In other words, the company should work toward establishing optimal practice conditions where the interests of employee-patients are not subordinate to those of the corporation.

NOTES

1. 64 ALR2d 1108.

2. 210 NC 756 (1936).

3. William L. Prosser, *The Law of Torts* (St. Paul: West Publishing, 1971), p. 344.

4. Pub.L. 91-596.

5. 29 CRF 1910:151.

6. 29 CRF 1910:1005 (g) (1), Regulations for 4,4'-Methylene bis (2-chloroaniline). Separate regulations are developed for various cancer-causing agents.

7. Edward A. Klein, "Warning: The Workplace May Be Hazardous to Your Health," *Trail Magazine*, November 1976, p. 34.

8. Harry Dahl, "The Inter-Relationship between Law and Medicine in Workmen's Compensation: A Comparative Guide for Physicians," *Cal Western Law Review* 12:25 (1975–76).

9. Stephen Altman, "Growing Pains: A Portrait of Developing Occupational Safety and Health in America," *Job Safety and Health*, August 1976, p. 24.

10. *Cox v. City of Milwaukee*, Workmen's Compensation Division, State of Wisconsin, August 15, 1975.

11. 253 SW2d 165 (1952).

12. 148 SE2d 548 (1966).

13. 251 IOWA 375 (1960).

14. 233 A2d 126 (1967).

15. 350 MASS 675 (1966).

16. 261 MICH 156 (1933).

17. 200 NYS 235 (1923).

18. 233 A2d 126 (1967).

19. 302 NE2d 580 (1972).

20. 40 ALR3d 1072.

21. 309 NE2d 420 (1974).

22. 16 ALR3d 564.

23. 45 NEB 570 (1895).

24. *Gosnell v. Southern Railroad Co.* 202 NC 234 (1932).

25. Ibid., §4(b).

26. Ibid.

27. 55 CA1 APP 734 (1921).

28. 212 SW 88 (1919).

29. *Jines v. General Electric Co.* 303 F2d 76 (1962).

30. 121 SE 174 (1924).

31. 33 ILL2d 326 (1965); *Gonzales v. Nork* CAL SUPER CT Sacramento Co. Docket no. 228-566. (1973).

32. See Richard L. Peck, "Peer Review, Courtesy Goodyear Tire & Rubber," *Medical Economics*, April 4, 1977, p. 31.

33. 22 SW2d 602 (1929).

34. 292 NYS 339 (1937).

35. 16 ALR3d 564.

36. 122 F.Supp. 899 (1954).

37. 158 F2d 973 (1947).

38. *Betesh v. U.S.* 400 F. Supp. 238 (1974).

39. Restatement of contracts 2d §90.

40. Perillo Calamari, *Contracts* (St. Paul: West Publishing, 1970), pp. 180–187.

41. Ibid., chapter 14.

42. See Calamari, op. cit., p. 273.

43. 20 TEX CIV APP 642 (1899).

44. *Ulbrich v. Boone County Coal* 16 PaD&C 315 (1931).

45. 129 CAL APP2d 482 (1954).

46. 230 CAL APP2d 960 (1964).

47. 158 F2d 973 (1947).

48. 302 NE2d 580 (1972).

49. 69 ALR2d 1213.

50. *Union Carbide and Carbon Corp. v. Stapleton* 237 F2d 229 (1956).

51. CAL SUPER CT, Contra Costa Co. Docket no. 11603, N.1 (1973).

52. 369 SW2d 705 (1973).

53. 183 NYS2d 351 (1959).

54. Ibid.

55. 503 P2d 1366 (1972).

56. 277 P2d 444 (1954).

57. 503 P2d 1366 (1972).

Economic Implications of Employer-Provided Health Care

Alan C. Monheit

18

The negative impact of employee ill health upon the economy is strikingly evident in the number of workdays lost, which has averaged a workweek per employee-year over the postwar era,[1] and in estimates of the resulting loss in goods and services. One estimate holds that a reduction in absenteeism of one day per employee-year would add $10 billion to the gross national product.[2] Poor employee health leads also to disruption of production schedules, and in some cases to recruitment and training costs for replacement workers. Indeed, formal research by economists has found health status a significant determinant of various components of labor supply and of increased productivity.[3]

Perhaps one of the most glaring consequences of employee ill health is the rising cost of health care fringe benefits. Combined employer and employee contributions to health benefits are now more than twenty-five times their 1950 levels, reflecting larger benefits paid, more workers covered, broadened scope of services offered, and inflated medical care prices.* Both management and labor have expressed concern over these increases, and both parties have sought greater control over employee health status and utilization of health services through review of insurance claims, support of HMOs, and direct provision health services and health education.[4]

Expansion of the corporate clinic (originally developed to deliver occupational health care) to provide preventive and primary health care to employees has been suggested as one way in which the firm can monitor and influence employee health and ultimately, perhaps, reduce its health care expenditures. This proposal merits analysis in economic terms to determine its appropriateness and likelihood of success. Obviously, the most telling approach would be a rigorous cost-benefit analysis, but this is precluded by lack of the necessary data. However, several other economic concepts assist in evaluating, if only in general terms, the advisability of offering expanded services through in-house corporate clinics.

The Firm as A Provider of Health Services

The greatly changed stake of employers in the health of their employees as a result of benefit programs has stimulated management interest in the question, whether, and in what degree, it may be to its advantage to fill some of the gaps and weaknesses in community health care by initiating, or broadening in-house programs of primary care.[5]

Although management may have displayed an interest in directly providing health care services to employees, evidence from the early 1970s fails to disclose any substantial dollar commitments.** Expenditures for this purpose appear to be only a fraction of the total spent for health insurance and disability benefits. Perhaps, one would hope, this reflects an unwillingness to commit resources without careful consideration of alternative clinic service programs, or until existing in-house programs of primary care and health education have been evaluated.

In the absence of a definitive evaluation, we may still consider the appropriateness of health care in terms of two economic concepts: the notion of "externalities" or unaccounted social "costs" arising as a by-product of com-

*In 1950, less than half of all wage and salary workers were covered for hospitalization, surgical, and regular medical expenses; by 1974 over two-thirds of such workers were covered. Less than 1 percent of wage and salary workers had major medical expense insurance as a fringe benefit in 1952, but by 1974 a third of such workers had secured coverage. Health contributions and benefits paid experienced their greatest rise during the 1950s and maintained a double-digit rate of growth throughout the 1960s, accelerating slightly during 1970–1974. See Alfred M. Skolnik, "Twenty-Five Years of Employee Benefit Plans," *Social Security Bulletin* 39:3-2 (September 1976).

**In a 1971 survey of 585 firms employing 500 or more workers, the Conference Board found little change in industry commitment over the proceeding decade. 1971 median expenditures on in-house care per employee were about $11 with over 60 per cent of firms surveyed spending $15 or less. (Note, however, that the survey would fail to capture any rise in expenditures during the mid-1970s). Expenditures were found to correlate to some extent with various firm and worker characteristics (see Lusterman, op. cit.)

pany operation, and the notion of investment in "human capital". The first would treat work-related ill health as an actual "cost" of production, which is "paid" entirely by the employee unless the firm assumes the "cost" by providing care (or taking preventive measures). The second would treat the provision of care as a form of capital expenditure, whose expected returns (increased labor productivity, averted replacement cost, and so on) would be weighed against alternative investment opportunities (both human and nonhuman).

To the degree that employee ill health results from a firm's operations, there exist costs of production beyond those considered by the firm in its profit-maximizing calculations. If these costs are not somehow "paid," the firm is not *socially* efficient, however privately efficient it may be,* and labor will bear these costs in the form of illness and loss of income. As long as there is a pool of readily available workers, little or no replacement cost, and no legal responsibility for harm befalling employees, firms will have little incentive to assume these costs by improving job safety, providing medical care, or adjusting output levels.** The establishment of legal liability for social costs may encourage firms to invest in safety and medical services, *if* the cost of that investment is below the expected cost of violating the legal mandate. Inclusion of social costs in profit calculations would yield a more socially efficient level of output, but firms have historically ignored these costs and not implemented health and safety standards—unless compulsion was applied. The establishment of legal liability and penalty structures represents an effort to use quasi-market incentives to induce firms to recognize social costs. However, such imperfections as the difficulty of establishing liability for a particular instance of employee ill-health have led to a more direct, regulatory approach.[6] The health and safety standards in the Occupational Safety and Health Act (OSHAct) and insurance schemes such as no-fault Workmen's Compensation serve to partially shift costs from the employees to the firm, forcing it to assume costs—dictated by efficiency and equity—that employers generally fail to assume independently.

However, if firms perceive that returns emanate from investments in employee health, incentives will exist for them to make such investments voluntarily. "Human capital" investments have usually been discussed in the context of on-the-job training, but the same principles apply to investments in employee health through the provision of health services. Like any investment, firms will evaluate health services in terms of whether the expected rate of

---

*In economic terms, the socially efficient level of production is established when the marginal benefits from the last unit of output produced equal the full marginal social costs of producing that unit. This is entirely consistent with firm profit maximization since prices determined in competitive markets generally capture these factors. However, additional social costs may be created by production (externalities associated with pollution, accidents, and so on) that the market fails to reflect.

**Incentives can, however, be supplied through bargaining. If all available workers are aware of the danger, the firm may be induced to either pay higher wages to compensate for the risk, provide medical services, or improve job safety as a condition of employment. Alternatively, if a pool of replacement workers unaware of the danger is available, current workers may seek to "bribe" employers by offering to accept lower wages in exchange for improved job safety or medical services. For a detailed description of a number of alternative solutions based upon the liability and asset position of the firm see D. E. Williamson, Douglas G. Olson, and August Ralston, "Externatities, Insurance, and Disability Analysis" *Economica* (August 1967) 235–253.

return will exceed the returns from alternative dollar investments. The expected returns of health services might include increased worker productivity (through enhanced physical and mental capacities and reduction of workdays lost) and savings of the costs incurred from employee illness. These include search, training, and other costs of replacement, losses resulting from disruption of production, and future increments in health insurance premiums.* In addition, if in-house medical services are seen by employees as a valuable convenience or if they result in strong relationships between employee-patients and physicians, the firm may accrue some savings from reduced labor turnover. Firms may thus voluntarily apply resources to health care programs, as a result of the usual considerations governing any capital expenditure.

A closer examination of the nature of this investment does reveal, however, some complexities that may affect its attractiveness. One of these arises from the nature of human capital and of the returns that emanate from health care investments. Corporate investment in physical capital bestows ownership and hence rights to whatever returns are forthcoming. Human capital, on the other hand, cannot be owned by the firm, and its enjoyment of returns is subject to far greater uncertainty, for workers may leave employment, retire, or suddenly expire. Furthermore, there is considerable uncertainty as to whether returns actually emanate from various kinds of health expenditures and as to the firm's ability to capture them. Broad application of multiphasic screening, for example, has been criticized for its costs and for lack of demonstrable improvements in health status.[7]** Similarly, the efficacy of annual physical examinations has been seriously questioned.† If health status largely reflects life style, how far can the firm commit itself to effectuating change? Health education programs and information may be relatively inexpensive to offer, but the costs of getting workers to comply may be prohibitive. Finally, the elapsed time between expenditures on employee health and the receipt of returns is extremely difficult to reckon, thereby adding to the uncertainty of the investment. Such factors clearly diminish the attractiveness of this form of capital expenditure and suggest some sharing of its cost between firm and employee.

Joint responsibility for health care costs is also suggested by other human capital considerations, although no clear guidelines are provided as to relative shares. If we consider training for a moment, it is clear that human capital investments may either enhance productivity solely within a firm, in which

---

*One could also include among averted costs the possible penalties from noncompliance with medical standards required by OSHAct and any savings in reduced Workmen's Compensation payments.

**Work by Collen at Kaiser-Permanente failed to show significantly different rates of hospitalization attributable to screening. In fairness, however, the payoff to screening may be considerably improved if directed at high-risk groups. See "Economic Impact of Preventive Medicine," op. cit.

†In work by Collen at Kaiser over a seven-year period, no significant differences were disclosed in deaths, chronic disease, or disability and time lost between those having periodic examinations and those examined at their own inclination. "Except for the detection of hypertension and a handful of abnormalities, current data indicate that the periodic health exam, even when complemented by the multiphasic profile, is a costly indulgence that does little to insure health." Richard Spark, "The Case Against Regular Physicals," New York Times, July 25, 1976, p. VI–41.

case it should be financed by that firm, or it may impart skills that raise worker productivity in all firms, in which case it should be financed by the workers. Workers would be unwilling to invest in firm-specific training because loss of employment would entail loss of returns to their investment. Similarly, employers would avoid investment in generally applicable skills because returns would be lost if a worker moved to another firm.[8] In hybrid cases where both general and firm-specific characteristics are imparted, costs would be shared since some returns are captured by the firm and others by the worker in the form of the enhanced market value of his services. Health care investments constitute a hybrid case in the sense that returns accrue to firms providing care, are transferable to other firms, and benefit the employee both at work and in leisure. However, since no particular skill has been imparted, it remains unclear how the market will value the receipt of health services on the part of a worker or what a worker would be willing to invest for the future returns of such services. As a result, one should not expect either the firm or the worker to finance completely a comprehensive array of health services. Contributions from both should be required and, since market signals are unusually unclear on the "value" imparted, relative shares should be determined through negotiation.

If a firm should decide to provide medical care on a scale that encompasses preventive and primary care, it has by definition become involved in joint production of medical care along with its primary product. While economists have developed a theory of joint production that suggests that firms will produce both commodities in proportion to their relative costs and market prics, it does not apply well to the production of medical care. Corporate medical care is produced not to be old but to enhance labor productivity and avert illness-related costs. As a result, objective evaluations by the market concerning the appropriate level and scope of services are lacking. For example, it is uncertain whether a firm's health insurance expenditures will respond favorably to efforts to monitor employee health, and only a weak relationship has been found between changes in injury and disease rates and Workmen's Compensation premiums and benefits paid.[9] Thus it remains debatable whether the health services produced by the firm will be sufficient to deal with employee health problems.*

A second implication arising from the concept of joint production involves the scope and quality of medical services provided. Production of medical care entails diverting resources from a firm's primary commodity; and since high quality care usually requires greater resources, proportionately more of the primary commodity will be forgone. As a result, the firm will be susceptible to internal debates regarding trade-offs between cost and scope or quality reminiscent of the larger external controversy. One might expect, for example, pressures to develop from employee groups for internal quality assurance programs. Furthermore, variation in resources available to firms will

*Some skeptical views of corporate health programs on the part of both management and labor are reported in Lusterman, op. cit., chapter 2.

certainly be reflected in levels of quality, and may therefore perpetuate existing disparities in the quality of health services available to the work force.

Corporate involvement in joint production might also raise legal issues (see chapter 17 by Blum). Concern has been expressed, particularly by labor groups, that confidentiality of medical records may be violated when the physician is employed by the firm.* However, if the firm is to secure returns from its health care investments it must have access to information concerning employee health status; otherwise its ability to evaluate current and future health expenditures will be seriously impaired. Hence contractual agreements regarding access to medical records must be established, but this process may arouse the mistrust of employees and thereby negate efforts to establish the in-house medical program. It should also be noted that employers may find themselves faced with liability for malpractice occurring in their clinics. To the degree that such potential liability increases premiums for general insurance or Workmen's Compensation protection, the savings anticipated from the provision of services will be reduced.

In considering the potential advantages to the firm and to society of expanding corporate health services, I have expressed a number of reservations about whether firms would or should voluntarily commit resources beyond those required for occupational health and safety. These reservations are based on the nature of the expected returns (not firm-specific and not owned by the firm), on the lack of information about the impact of care on a firm's health-related and other costs, on the difficulties of determining adequate levels and quality of care, and on the associated costs of malpractice liability and of establishing access to medical records. It would be possible, however, for a firm to seek to justify provision of health care not for its own benefit, but as a gratuitous benefit for its employees. It would be useful, therefore, to explore in economic terms the impact of corporate health services on employee welfare.

Corporate Health Services' Impact on Employee Welfare

It may seem obvious that health care benefits extended by firms to their employees, through either health insurance plans or direct provision, improve employee welfare. However, before a complete and unambiguous endorsement is rendered, one should examine the impact such programs may have on employee income and purchasing patterns, as well as the ultimate "incidence" of program costs, that is, who actually pays for corporate health services.

The impact of nonvoluntary plans (such as health benefits, excise taxes, subsidies) on individual welfare can usually be seen in terms of changes in income and consumption opportunities.* In this case, one would compare the

---

*Corporate physicians have identified confidentiality as a potential problem. See Lusterman, op. cit., p. 19.

**My assessment skirts the issue of impact upon health status because insufficient data exist for conclusions to be drawn.

positions of a person who purchases medical services and any other commodity before and after the imposition of a particular health plan. The points raised should illustrate the difficulty of making conclusive statements regarding individual welfare.

In the absence of a plan, the individual is free to select any combination of medical services (M) and other commodities (X) whose cost is within his total income. A plan is then imposed offering "free" primary care and other care at a reduced price.* A lump-sum payment is necessary for participation, to be paid directly or indirectly by the employee.** Naturally, the individual will be unable to spend for X the amount of the participation fee; after this is paid, however, his use of primary care will have no effect on his other consumption, and his use of further services at reduced rates will have less effect on his other consumption than would a comparable choice of medical services before joining the plan (when their full market price had to be paid).

The impact of this plan on the person's welfare depends upon his relative preferences for medical services and other commodities. If he has a preference for medical services, he gains, since he can now consume more M without reducing his purchases of X. If, however, his preference is for other commodities, his welfare is reduced, since after paying the participation fee he has less available to spend for X. The degree of loss or gain in these two cases will obviously depend on the size of the fee and the amount of the copayment for services beyond primary care. The scope of the services included in the free category will affect gainers—the more free care, the greater their gains; but those whose welfare is reduced will be affected differentially according to the strength of their preference for X in relation to M. If no medical services are desired, their welfare is unaffected by variations in the free care offered; if some M is desired, their losses would be reduced or they could even become gainers as the scope of free services is increased. However, unless we know consumer tastes for medical services in relation to other commodities, we cannot assess the over-all impact of a health plan on consumer welfare. But knowing that some employees may suffer decreased welfare under a plan should discourage endorsement of corporate health services as an unqualified benefit to employees.

This example may be viewed as an overly restrictive description of the effects on employee welfare of corporate health care plans. After all, I have not included the option of health plans available outside the firm; nor have I explained why corporate plans exist if the potential for reducing welfare is present. As to the former, the corporate plans are probably the most relevant comparisons with the no-plan situation. The economies of group purchasing,

---

*If a third level of care is established beyond the copayment category for which full payment is required, the results would not be altered.

**If the employer pays the cost of participating and does not shift the incidence to the employees, then employees clearly gain since they can consume more of either or both M and X under the plan, assuming that preplan purchases of M were not zero. If the employee purchased no health services before the plan, that is, if he devoted his entire income to X, then the imposition of the plan would not further increase his ability to buy X, but would of course increase his ability to consume primary care while holding consumption of X constant. The critical issue here is the ultimate incidence of the participation fee. This is explored below.

tax advantages, and employer contributions should reduce the price of such a plan below that for similar protection purchased independently. More importantly, employees may have no choice between participation and nonparticipation: the cost of tailoring a plan to individual employee preferences would be prohibitive. As to the reasons for existence of plans that could reduce welfare, it has been suggested that the plans defined through collective bargaining may reflect the preferences of the "median" worker in the firm, but plans defined by employers may be somewhat more occupation-specific.[10] Thus it is possible for some employees to suffer losses in welfare, to the extent that their preferences are not met and compensation through wage adjustments is not feasible.

The critical issue in the above example and in any welfare analysis of employee health care programs—and one that can easily be overlooked—is who ultimately pays their cost. Health programs are frequently seen only as fringe benefits, which seems to connote additional income-in-kind that is paid for by the employer beyond whatever employee contributions are required. However, "fringe benefit" may be a misnomer if the firm has agreed to pay for such services on a per employee basis and if the labor contract is flexible regarding wage and employment-level adjustments. Mitchell and Vogel have drawn an analogy on the issue of incidence between health insurance benefits financed on a per employee basis and a payroll tax:

> Both economic theory and empirical research on payroll taxes strongly suggest that employees bear most, if not all of the burden of such taxes by receiving lower cash wages than they would in the absence of the tax. Health insurance "fringe benefits" are formally similar to payroll taxes, but with the additional consideration that they are established by agreement between the individual firm and its employees and that benefits from the insurance are generally consumed as medical services during the period of employment.[11]

Corporate health care services financed in a like manner may be readily included in the comparison, and the ultimate incidence of their cost depends upon the ease with which the firm can adjust wages and/or employment. This is not to say that the concern expressed by firms over the rise in their contributions to health care plans is largely illusory. Rather, it is only to suggest that such concern ultimately reflects labor cost increases not easily justified by productivity levels, combined with limited ability to shift these costs. For a profit-maximizing firm in a competitive environment, these are certainly not minor considerations.

The wage offered by a firm may contain dollar and nondollar components. If the latter are provided (for instance, in the form of medical care), the firm will be forced under competitive condiions to adjust the monetary component of wages downward by a compensating dollar value so that total wage paymens reflect the value of employee productivity. Failure to so adjust would negate the profit-maximizing or cost-minimizing goal established by the firm. If employees recognize in-kind services as a component of their wage, the adjustment can be made. It is in this sense that an employee properly bears the cost of "fringe" benefits.* If workers fail to recognize "fringe" health service benefits as a form of compensation (and view them, for instance, as a safety requirement), and even if the employment contract precludes off-setting wage adjustments, then labor will still bear a portion of the program costs. Adjustment can take the form of reduced employment levels, depending upon the ease with which overtime hours and capital can be substituted.** However, if the employment contract provides little room for either wage or employment adjustments to compensate for the cost of fringe benefits offered or for their uncontrollable growth, then employers will find themselves bearing a disproportionate share of the cost. This may well be the current situation faced by employers with respect to health insurance premiums, with their competitive positions barring attempts to recapture costs through product price increases.

There are, in addition, equity considerations that go beyond these implications of economic productivity theory. If employee ill health results from conditions of employment, the cost of health services should not be viewed as a nonmonetary component of wages, but should instead be borne by employers as a part of the full social cost of production. If, however, ill health arises from employee life style, corporate health services should be recognized as a nonmonetary component of income and their cost borne by employees. Finally, if health services constitute an investment in human capital, both should contribute. This is not to say that such demarcations are easy or practical to make— rather, it suggests that equity requires, at a minimum, sharing the cost.

Alternatives to Employer-Provided Health Services

I have taken a rather skeptical view of the firm's potential as a direct provider of health care. This is not to say, however, that industry has little to contribute to a reshaping of our overall health care delivery system. Industry *can* play an integral part by extending its managerial skills to the health care sector and by creating incentives for employees to utilize the more efficient providers.

In general, the economic problems of our health care system result from our population's health status and the mismanagement of existing health services. In altering health status, health care policy may play only a limited role (as in structuring incentives to alter life style) since status is intimately related to behavioral, environmental, and genetic factors. The problem of poor management, however, leads to a misallocation of existing health care resources: overutilization and expansion of hospital services and facilities, excessive reliance on physician services, failure to extend the role of auxiliary

*A detailed analysis of the incidence of payroll taxes for social security contribution by employers is provided by John A. Brittain, "The Incidence of Social Security Payroll Taxes," *American Economic Review* 61:110–125 (March 1971). The basic arguments above are drawn from his contribution.

**Ronald G. Ehrenberg provides some evidence that overtime hours will be increased as the ratio of supplementary benefits to the overtime wage rate increases. See *Fringe Benefits and Overtime Behavior* (Lexington, Mass.: D. C. Heath, 1971).

health personnel, and infusion of costly health care technology, to name a few. These abuses have been encouraged by the nonprofit nature of health care institutions, by the unbridled reliance on fee-for-service medical care, and by third-party financing. It is in this area that the management and negotiating skills of industry have perhaps their greatest potential.

Specific uses for industry's managerial expertise have been suggested.[12] Participating on hospital boards of trustees and in health systems planning agencies, assisting Blue Cross and Blue Shield review boards, aiding health care institutions with their financial systems, establishing reimbursement policies and charges with insurers, and negotiating cost-sharing incentives with labor groups are all potentially valuable roles.[13] In addition, industry can lend support to the design and operation of prepaid health plans (HMOs), which have been generally recognized as reducing health care costs (primarily through limiting unnecessary hospitalization). Given the federal mandate in support of HMOs (an act of Congress in 1973 and further amendments in 1976), industry might encourage their growth by helping to prepare the necessary marketing and feasibility studies, by coordinating and consolidating support from insurance, medical, and other interests in the community, and by helping to secure the required start-up capital.[14] Such a stance would require a change in the passive role generally taken by firms toward the manner in which health care is delivered.*

Firms may also assist HMOs by encouraging employees to enroll. Economists have found that the time costs associated with gaining access to medical care (waiting and travel times) can be significant impediments. Preliminary work by McGuire, who studied the choice made by Yale University employees between traditional Blue Cross–Blue Shield coverage and a university-sponsored HMO, found that distance from the plan significantly discouraged entry.[15] To counter such an effect, employers could subsidize the time during which workers seek care. Furthermore, since the premium required for HMO membership is likely to be somewhat higher than those of the more traditional insurance options (reflecting the increased scope of care required under federal legislation), employers may act to reduce the disparity by sharing more of the cost or by providing lobbying support to amend federal requirements and thus make HMOs more competitive. Finally, by studying the characteristics of their work force, firms may assist in designing attractive HMO plans. Work by Berki et al., for example, suggests that younger people with families who are new to an area prefer closed-panel HMO organization, while families with longer residence in a community and stronger physician ties would prefer to join their physician in open-panel or "foundation-type" organizations.[16]** Awareness of such characteristics could significantly aid the HMOs' efforts to secure the

---

*The 1971 Conference Board survey notes a number of issues firms must confront before lending their support, but survey findings reveal that some firms have entered "a middle ground of encouragement and of financial, managerial, and technical support for HMO development." Lusterman, op. cit., pp. 61–66.

**Foundation models are prepaid plans that reimburse on a fee-for-service basis and permit independent practices to continue. Such plans would generally require less start-up capital. (See chapters 1 by Spies and 10 by Himler.)

required membership. All these suggestions involve certain costs to be borne by the firm, but they are made in light of evidence suggesting potential cost savings from use of this mode of health care delivery.

I would like to mention one last but equally significant role for industry. Firms can provide a natural laboratory where the requisite data may be obtained to assess the impact of various efforts aimed at securing employee health. Further work is certainly required to ascertain the costs and benefits of various preventive health care activities, the incentives required for employee HMO participation, and the feasibility and success of HMOs themselves—are they ultimately less costly or, as some critics have suggested, do they merely serve an unrepresentative population? By providing research opportunities for social scientists and health policymakers, industry can help resolve these and other difficult policy issues.

NOTES

1. *Statistical Abstract of the United States*, U.S. Department of Commerce, 1976, table 138, p. 88.

2. A 1965 estimate cited in Nicholas Ashford, *Crisis in the Workplace* (Cambridge, Mass.: MIT Press, 1976).

3. Michael Grossman and Lee Benham, "Health, Hours, and Wages," in *The Economics of Health and Medical Care*, ed. Marc Perlman (New York: John Wiley, 1974); and Richard Scheffler and George Iden, "The Effect of Disability on Labor Supply," *Industrial and Labor Relations Review* 28:122-132 (October 1974).

4. See "Employer Health Care Benefits: Labor-Management Innovations in Controlling Cost," *Federal Register* 41:10298-10326 (September 17, 1976); and Seymour Lusterman, *Industry Roles in Health Care* (New York: The Conference Board, 1974).

5. Lusterman, op. cit.

6. See Ashford, op. cit., pp. 18–20, 333–359.

7. See "Economic Impact of Preventive Medicine," in *Preventive Medicine USA*, Task Force Reports sponsored by the John E. Fogarty International Center for Advanced Study in the Health Sciences, National Institutes of Health, and the American College of Preventive Medicine (New York: Prodist, 1976), pp. 696–697; Marvin M. Kristein et al., "Health Economics and Preventive Care," *Science* 195:460 (February 4, 1977); "Theory, Practice, and Application of Prevention in Personal Health Services," in *Preventive Medicine USA*, op. cit., pp. 30–36; and Charles E. Phelps, "Benefit/Cost Analysis of Quality Assurance Programs," in *Quality Assurance in Health Care*, ed. R. H. Egdahl and P. M. Gertman (Germantown, Md.: Aspen Systems Corp., 1976), pp. 319–324, for discussions of the cost-benefit relationships of selected preventive health services.

8. See Gary S. Becker, *Human Capital*, 2nd ed. (New York: National Bureau of Economic Research, 1975).

9. Ashford, op. cit., p. 318.

10. Gerald Goldstein and Mark Pauly, "Group Health Insurance as a Public Good," in *The Role of Health Insurance in the Health Services Sector*, ed. Richard N. Rossett (New York: National Bureau of Economic Research, 1976).

11. Bridger M. Mitchell and Ronald Vogel, "Health and Taxes: An Assessment of the Medical Deduction," *Southern Economic Journal* 41:664-665 (April 1975).

12. See, for example, Irving Leveson, *Medical Care Costs*, Corporate Environmental Program Research Memorandum no. 29 (Croton-on-Hudson, N.Y.: Hudson Institute, July 1976).

13. See "Employee Health Care Benefits," op. cit., for specific examples of the latter.

14. See Ibid. and Verne C. Johnson, "Roles for Business in HMO Development: Lessons of the Twin Cities Project," in *Health Care Issues for Industry*, ed. Seymour Lusterman (New York: The Conference Board, 1974), pp. 78–84.

15. Thomas G. McGuire, "Choice of Membership in a Prepaid Group Practice," unpublished, Boston University Department of Economics, 1976.

16. S. E. Berki et al., "Enrollment Choices in a Multi-HMO Setting: The Roles of Health Risk, Financial Vulnerability, and Access to Care," *Medical Care* 15:95-114 (February 1977).

Index